The Resilient Physician:

Effective Emotional Management for Doctors and Their Medical Organizations

Wayne M. Sotile, PhD, and Mary O. Sotile, MA

The Resilient Physician:
Effective Emotional Management for
Doctors and Their Medical Organizations

This book is for informational purposes only. It is not intended to constitute legal or financial advice. If legal, financial, or other professional advice is required, the services of a competent professional should be sought.

Additional copies of this book may be ordered by calling 800 621-8335.
Secure on-line orders can be taken at www.ama-assn.org/catalog.
Mention product number OP209801.

ISBN 1-57947-243-5
BP37:0100-01:10/01

To physicians everywhere, the unsung heroes of our culture. We admire and appreciate what you and your families do to create safe spaces for the rest of us.

Wayne M. Sotile, PhD, and **Mary O. Sotile, MA,** are codirectors of Sotile Psyhological Associates, PLLC and Real Talk, Inc, in Winston-Salem, North Carolina, where Wayne also serves as Director of Psychological Services at the Wake Forest University Cardiac Rehabilitation Program. They have authored six books, including *The Medical Marriage: Sustaining Healthy Relationships for Physicians and Their Families* (AMA Press: 2000) and *Beat Stress Together: The BEST Way to a Passionate Marriage, a Healthy Family, and a Productive Life* (Wiley: 1999; audio: 1999). The Sotiles' work on well-being for high-performing people and collegiality and collaboration in the medical workplace has been featured in the professional literature and in the international popular media, including national television. Their column, "The Medical Marriage Journey," is a regular feature in the AMA-Alliance's publication, *The Alliance Today.* The Sotiles serve as consultants to numerous medical practices and hospitals, and they have provided individualized assessment and counseling to nearly 1,000 physicians. They are also among the most sought after speakers and workshop leaders, having presented more than 1,500 keynotes to gatherings of medical professionals.

More information about the Sotiles and advice for medical families is available from their web site, www.Sotile.com. Contact them at wsotile@attglobal.net or at 1396 Old Mill Circle, Winston-Salem, NC 27103.

ACKNOWLEDGMENTS

We thank the many people who foster our own resilience through their personal and professional support:

- The great folks at the American Medical Association Press, especially Suzanne Fraker, Anne Serrano, Patrick Dati, J.D. Kinney, Rosalyn Carlton, and Ronnie Summers—for believing in us and in our work.

- The gracious and heroic members of the American Medical Association Alliance—for being the original and sustaining beacons of hope regarding the issues that matter most for physicians and their families.

- The many medical organizations and hospital systems that continue to allow us the privilege of working with them to promote resilient medical cultures.

- The many pharmaceutical companies, medical practices, medical schools, and hospitals that support educational programs that promote physician resilience—for allocating resources that truly make a difference.

- Our wonderful colleagues at Sotile Psychological Associates—for helping to create the best, most pleasant practice we know.

- And, as always, to our daughters, Rebecca and Julia—for trusting and loving us enough to still let us in on your secrets. You are the true sources of our resilience.

CONTENTS

INTRODUCTION

"**P**ower is having control over one's own life."[1] This said, consider the lives of most physicians today. Busy medical professionals have always lived pressure-packed lives. That's nothing new. But, historically, physicians also enjoyed high levels of control. They ruled their workplaces, they typically were supported by a stay-at-home spouse, and they enjoyed high levels of autonomy. In other words, their professional lives were characterized by high demand and *high control.*

How times have changed! Physicians today face excessive workloads and the mandate to "speed up"—to do more work, learn new skills, and adjust to an endless stream of changes that are not in their direct control. At the same time, physicians' personal lives have been reshaped. The typical medical family today has changed dramatically in both form and function.[2] Now, more than ever before, being a physician means encountering high-demand/*low-control* stress, both at work and at home.[3]

As control is stripped from high-powered copers, a negative emotional chain reaction often results. The attitudes and emotions of key players in any group tend to be "contagious."[4] When the leaders are optimistic, they tend to shape a group optimism; when leaders are resilient, the group tends to respond with resilience. However, when people in positions of authority mismanage their emotions, the negative consequences spread like viruses. An authority figure who shows such emotions as anger, depression, and agitation and attitudes such as cynicism, hostility, and suspiciousness can negatively affect every individual in his or her path. For many physicians, the strained relationships and loss of support that result from mismanagement of their emotions proves to be the final ingredient in a recipe for stress, dissatisfaction, and burnout.[5] High demand/low control is bad enough; high demand/low control/*low support* can be deadly.[6]

Our work as consultants to more than 400 medical organizations and as counselors to thousands of medical families has lead us to conclude that many physicians today are ill-equipped to handle the escalating tensions and complicated interpersonal

dynamics they face. Inadvertently, they become the source of negative emotional contagion, both at work and at home. The symptoms of this painful trap are not difficult to recognize. You know
you're in trouble if you:

- Find yourself chronically frustrated with medical colleagues or
  administrators whose actions complicate, rather than soothe,
  what stresses you.
- Find yourself working harder but feeling that you are
  accomplishing less.
- Find your colleagues criticize you for not working hard enough
  while your loved ones complain that you work too much.
- Find that your relationships with patients, colleagues, and
  loved ones are generally more stressful than soothing.

What is Effective Emotional Management and Why Is it Important?

For the past 25 years, we have worked as consultants and counselors to physicians, medical practices, and hospital systems in
the areas of conflict management, stress management, work—
family balance, and physician well-being. Much of our careers
have been devoted to learning the secrets of high-performing,
stress-hardy physicians and medical groups, those busy men and
women who manage to replace negative coping styles with positive ones. We wrote *The Resilient Physician* in order to share what
we have learned from these extraordinary copers.

This is a book filled with commonsense advice about how to
enhance physician well-being and stress resilience. We call our
model for stress-hardiness effective emotional management, or
EEM. This model is an amalgam of key points about stress
resilience gleaned from research and clinical experience. EEM
moves beyond traditional approaches in that it incorporates
strategies for identifying and managing two essential components
of stress management: Personality-based coping patterns and
relationship dynamics.

The material in this book is designed to help you to accomplish the following goals:

- Increase your coping range and flexibility
- Gain skills to better manage your emotions at work and home

- Decrease maladaptive acting-out of emotions, unconscious conflicts, and other destructive psychological patterns
- Increase your ability to manage yourself and others in times of crisis and conflict
- Improve your ability to balance work, family, and self

The skills necessary for EEM include:

- Honestly assessing your own coping patterns
- Taking responsibility for managing personality-based coping tendencies
- Managing attitudes that drive coping behaviors
- Disrupting maladaptive coping habits, including workaholism and other compulsions
- Treating your body/mind/spirit with respect
- Counteracting toxic emotions
- Learning to self-nurture with healthy pleasures
- Using positive interpersonal skills, like assertion, anger management, and principled conflict negotiation
- Employing realistic work-family balancing strategies

Why Bother?

If you learn to use these EEM skills, you can benefit in two ways: (1) You can avoid or eliminate the negative consequences that come with emotional *mismanagement;* and (2) you can gain positives, like greater collaboration with colleagues, cooperation from patients, and affection with loved ones.

But our call to physicians to learn to be effective emotional managers is not only about improving quality of life; EEM also makes good business sense. Research has documented that the way in which emotions are managed in the medical workplace has interpersonal consequences that influence productivity, morale, and outcomes. For example, developing positive teamwork has been found to be one of the most powerful organizational interventions to improving mental health in the workplace.[7] In addition, in the largest-ever patient satisfaction survey[8]—more than 1 million patients at 545 hospitals throughout the United States were surveyed—the 10 factors that correlated most highly with patient satisfaction were interpersonal factors.[5] Finally, a recent survey of 2,584 Canadian physicians found that major sources of satisfaction for both male and female physicians were the quality of their relationships with patients and colleagues.[9]

These findings and many others that will be reviewed in this book suggest that the true leadership challenge facing today's physicians is to develop ways to help medical organizations and medical families become positive interpersonal cultures.[10] This requires the ability to communicate well, develop and maintain teamwork, and use personal emotional management skills.[11] *The Resilient Physician* is intended to help you do just that.

Overview

In this book, we explain how managing your emotions is a key to personal stress-resilience and to building successful organizations. We teach you how to effectively and flexibly deal with others. And we teach you how to manage your own stress reactions and how to respond to others when they are stressed.

Section I focuses on personal assessment and management strategies. The truth about stress and work for physicians is explored in Chapter 1. Chapter 2 presents a series of self-assessment scales and frameworks that can help you to better understand your stress patterns and potential for work addiction. The chapter also offers practical stress management advice. In Chapter 3, we present a compassionate look at the psychology of today's physicians, emphasizing coping rather than psychopathology. Chapter 4 presents 10 keys to stress resilience. In Chapter 5, we present practical guidelines for balancing work and family life.

In Section II, we shift focus to understanding and managing relationships in the medical workplace. Chapter 6 provides an overview of conflict management styles and assessment strategies. Chapter 7 discusses the costs of mismanaged anger and remedies for it. Chapter 8 specifies models for effective conflict negotiation, and Chapter 9 addresses the special topic of the disruptive physician. Chapter 10 discusses listening and communication skills. Strategies for coping with change are presented in Chapter 11. Chapter 12 addresses the special coping challenges faced by medical students and residents. And we close with Chapter 13's discussion of how collaborative efforts can help to create positive interpersonal cultures in the medical workplace.

Throughout *The Resililent Physician* we present simple inventories that can be reproduced and used to assess individual coping styles and interpersonal dynamics in medical practices, hospital settings, and medical families. It is our hope that these tools will be used in the spirit of encouragement and support that we intend.

Research has suggested that the majority of physicians would welcome informal counseling regarding stress and relationship issues in the workplace.[12] This finding certainly matches our experiences as consultants to hospitals and medical practices: With rare exception, even the skeptics respond positively to workshops and seminars that teach tangible, commonsense coping strategies that are respectful of the medical culture. We sincerely believe that following our guidelines can help you to become more stress-resilient and a better source of resilience for others. If you already enjoy positive coping and happy relationships, perhaps our words will echo the sage advice of psychologist and philosopher William James: "We need not so much to be instructed as to be reminded."

References–Introduction

1. Farrell W. *Why Men Are The Way They Are*. New York, NY: Berkley Books; 1986.

2. Sotile WM, Sotile MO. *The Medical Marriage: Sustaining Healthy Relationships for Physicians and Their Families*. Chicago, Ill: American Medical Association; 2000.

3. Karasek R, Theorell T. *Healthy Work: Stress, Productivity, and the Reconstruction of Working Life*. New York, NY: Basic Books; 1990.

4. Weisinger H. *Anger at Work: Learning the Art of Anger Management on the Job*. New York, NY: William Morrow & Co; 1995.

5. Murphy LR. Organisational interventions to reduce stress in health care professionals. In: Firth-Cozens J, Payne R, eds. *Stress in Health Professionals: Psychological and Organisational Causes and Interventions*. New York, NY: John Wiley & Sons; 1999:149–162.

6. Jones F, Fletcher B. Job control and health. In: Sharbracq MJ, Winnibust JAM, Cooper CL, eds. *Handbook of Work and Health Psychology,* Chichester: Wiley; 1996.

7. Guzzo RA, Shea GP. Group performance and intergroup relations. In: Dunnette MD, Hough LM, eds. *Handbook of Industrial and Organisational Psychology*. Palo Alto, Calif: Consulting Psychologists Press; 1992:269–313.

8. Regrut B. *One Million Patients Have Spoken: Who Will Listen?* South Bend, Ind: Press, Ganey Associates; 1997.

9. Richardsen AM, Burke RJ. Occupational stress and job satisfaction among physicians: Sex differences. *Soc Sci Med.* 1991;33:1179–1187.

10. Sotile WM, Sotile MO. Conflict management, part 1: How to shape positive relationships in medical practices and hospitals. *The Physician Executive.* 1999;25:57–61.

11. Moss F, Paice E. Getting things right for the doctor in training. In: Firth-Cozens J, Payne R, eds. *Stress in Health Professionals: Psychological and Organisational Causes and Interventions*. New York, NY: John Wiley & Sons; 1999:203–218.

12. King MB, Cockcroft A, Gooch C. Emotional distress: Sources, effects and help sought. *J Royal Soc Med.* 1992;85:605–608.

Defining and Exploring Personal Assessment and Management Strategies

What *Really* Stresses Physicians

"Never have so many physicians worked so much for so little income and so little gratitude."

Sullivan and Buske[1] (p. 525)

What ever happened to the good old days? This is a question we often hear physicians ask, one that reflects a phenomenon worth noting.

The 1970s were years of high job and career satisfaction for physicians. In a 1973 survey of 2,700 physicians, 85.6% "had no doubt at all" about their career choice.[2] In those days of television shows like *Marcus Welby, M.D.*, physicians enjoyed unquestioned social esteem.

In the 1980s and 1990s, however, levels of physician satisfaction declined, as did overall social esteem for the profession. Gallup polls conducted by the American Medical Association in 1989 and 1990 showed that only 60% of physicians interviewed would definitely or probably enter medical school again.[3] Approximately 65% of physicians surveyed still report high levels of satisfaction with their work.[4,5] But the relative percentage of physicians who report *dissatisfaction* has grown considerably over the past decade.[6] In fact, by the late 1990s, approximately 37% of physicians polled stated that they were less satisfied than they were as recently as 5 years prior.[5] As the twentieth century drew to a close, Becker, the cynical curmudgeon played by Ted Danson in the popular television program of the same name, has replaced Marcus Welby.

This is important information. Research has indicated that chronic job strain may be dangerous to a physician's emotional and physical health.[7,8] Furthermore, decreased physician job satisfaction has been shown to correlate with increased employee

turnover rates, poor peer relations, and poor patient response.[9]
Specifically, patient populations treated by physicians who are
dissatisfied with their jobs have higher no-show rates, lower compliance rates, and low levels of reported satisfaction with the
quality of their medical care.[10] Higher physician job satisfaction,
on the other hand, has been shown to positively affect patients'
general adherence.[11] Clearly, when physicians are satisfied with
their jobs and in reasonable control of stress, both they *and* their
patients benefit.[12,13]

PHYSICIANS, BURNOUT, AND STRESS

Burnout is a state of physical, emotional, and mental exhaustion
that results from intense involvement with people over long periods of time in situations that are emotionally demanding.[14] One
manifestation of burnout is career dissatisfaction. But the more
than 4,400 publications on burnout[15] suggest that any combination
of the following seven symptom clusters can identify this syndrome:

- Distressed affect (eg, depressed mood, emotional exhaustion)
- Impaired cognitive processing (poor concentration)
- Elevated frequency of physical symptoms of stress (eg, head-
  aches, sleep disturbances)
- Impaired behavioral performance (eg, poor work performance)
- Loss of motivation for work (eg, loss of idealism)
- Interpersonal distress (irritability, dehumanization, indifference)
- Signs of organizational distress (eg, dissatisfaction, job
  turnover, low morale)

In its extreme form, burnout is signaled by physical depletion and
chronic fatigue, feelings of helplessness and hopelessness, and
negative attitudes toward self, work, life, and other people.
Clinical experience suggests that physicians who suffer burnout
tend to complain of a sense of futility and an inability to "bounce
back" as readily as usual. They feel that they work hard but do
not accomplish their goals; even after a weekend or day off from
work, their energies are not restored.

It is important to note that burnout tends to be job related and
situation specific, rather than pervasive. Burnout is not the same
as being generally overstressed, and it differs from depression in

that it is the final stage in the breakdown of coping reserves *specifically relative to work.*

ARE YOU SUFFERING FROM BURNOUT?

The most widely used scale for assessing burnout is the Maslach Burnout Inventory.[14] Using a series of 22 questions, this inventory assesses degrees of emotional exhaustion, depersonalization, and perceived personal accomplishment. A valid diagnosis of burnout requires that you formally take and score the Maslach Burnout Inventory[14] or an equivalent instrument. Here, we simply want to stimulate your thinking about your work attitudes and experiences and to give you an overview of the factors that can contribute to burnout.

You might be at risk of *emotional exhaustion* if you frequently:

- Find yourself emotionally drained from your work
- Feel depleted at the end of the workday
- Feel fatigued when you have to face another day of work
- Find work to be a strain
- Feel burned out from work
- Are frustrated with your work
- Believe that you are working too hard on your job
- Are strained by having to work with people
- Feel as though you are at the end of your rope

You might be at risk of suffering *depersonalization* if you frequently:

- Act as though you do not have compassion for patients and colleagues and tend to treat them as impersonal objects
- Become more callous toward people as a result of your job
- Find that work seems to be hardening you emotionally
- Act as though you are indifferent about what happens to people at work
- Feel blamed by people at work

You might be at risk of suffering a *diminished sense of personal accomplishment* if you frequently:

- Are losing empathy for others at work
- Are losing your effectiveness in dealing with the problems of other people at work
- Question whether your work really makes a difference in the lives of other people
- Are not very energetic
- Have difficulty creating a relaxed atmosphere at work
- Feel exhausted when you work closely with others
- Question whether you really accomplish anything worthwhile at work
- Are losing your ability to remain calm when dealing with emotional problems at work

Our effective emotional management (EEM) strategies can help prevent or ameliorate burnout. Start by flagging the factors that might put you at risk. In the remainder of this chapter, we discuss stressors that have historically been linked to physician burnout and present new ideas about what stresses today's physicians. We also introduce the EEM concepts for promoting physician resilience.

WHAT CAUSES PHYSICIAN BURNOUT?

For decades, we have assumed that physician burnout was caused by long work hours. Indeed, 3 times more physicians work 60 plus hours each week than any other profession.[16] But more recent research has clearly shown that the amount of time spent at work is but one of a combination of factors that may put you at risk. Despite the fact that the quality of research on burnout is often questionable, Schaufeli[17] noted that this literature emphasizes the importance of interplay among the following seven variables in determining burnout:

- Certain biographic characteristics (eg, younger age, little work experience)
- Personality factors that predispose one to high levels of anxiety or interpersonal conflict (eg, poor self-esteem, obsessiveness, social anxiety, dysthymia)

- Work-related attitudes that promote either unrealistic expectations, high perceived work stress, or low commitment to the organization
- General job stressors (eg, lack of autonomy, high workload, lack of feedback)
- Specific job stressors (eg, death and dying)
- Individual physical or mental health problems
- Organizational factors (eg, poor support staff, impaired organizational performance or morale)

McCranie and Brandsma[18] conducted a 25-year follow-up assessment of 440 practicing physicians in various specialties who had completed psychological testing upon entry into medical school. This study offered insights into what *does* and *does not* cause physician burnout. First, burnout did not associate with a variety of work-related factors, including medical specialty, practice arrangement, hours worked, and percentage of work time spent interacting with patients. The two factors that *did* correlate most strongly with burnout in the McCranie and Brandsma study were the physician's personality makeup and the degree of *perceived* job stress.

Personality Makeup

Clearly, physicians who are most at risk of burnout tend to show signs of vulnerability early in their careers. Especially at risk are those who begin their medical careers with traits of insecurity, low self-esteem, dependency, social anxieties, proneness to depression, a tendency to obsessively worry, low self-confidence, passivity, and social withdrawal.[18] However, it would be a mistake to assume that any student or physician who shows such characteristics is doomed to suffer burnout. As we discuss in Chapter 3, coping styles can be changed and vulnerable individuals can be helped to improve their levels of self-esteem and self-confidence.[19]

Perceived Work Stress

The most noteworthy observation in the McCranie and Brandsma[18] study is that the *perception* of job stress, rather than any set of objective characteristics of a physician's job, may cause

TABLE 1-1

Summary of Stress Research Conducted Prior to 1985

Study	Stressor Identified by Physician Sample
Krakowski[20]	Noncompliant, recalcitrant patients
	Dealing with dying patients or those not responding to treatment
	Interpersonal problems with colleagues and consultants
	Excessive paperwork
Mawardi[21]	Not enough personal free time
	Being on call
	Heavy workload
	For recent graduates: fears of mistakes, malpractice suits, and violent patients
Clarke et al[22]	Calls at night
	Excessive workload
	Difficult or dying patients
	Interpersonal conflicts
Anwar[23]	Keeping up with the medical literature
	Knowing enough
	Learning new skills and procedures
McCranie et al[24]	Time pressures
	Financial costs of practice
	Paperwork
	Interfacing with external regulatory agencies
Linn et al[25]	In academic medicine: salary limitations, publish-or-perish requirements

burnout. If this is so, a crucial question is, What do physicians find to be stressful about their jobs? Answers to this question have varied considerably over the past two decades. As noted in Table 1-1, research conducted prior to 1985 suggested a wealth of stressors, including workload issues, patient care issues, time pressures, and paperwork.[10]

Research in the 1990s added new dimensions to this list of perceived stressors. Complaints about paperwork and time demands persist, but many contemporary physicians perceive actual or feared losses and various types of interpersonal strife to be their major stressors. The following list summarizes the findings from a number of researchers[1,16,26,27] regarding what stresses physicians today:

- Concerns about competency
- Fears of medical practice lawsuits
- Changes in methods of reimbursement
- Increased paperwork
- Decreased income
- Government and insurance company regulations interfering with physician autonomy
- Deterioration of the physician–patient relationship
- Patients' unreasonable expectations of the health care system
- The responsibility inherent in the profession
- Conflict between career and family obligations
- Frustration with the hurdles in getting patients adequate consultant care

HAVE THINGS GOTTEN WORSE, NOT BETTER?

Regardless of their reasons, physicians today rate themselves as being more stressed than ever before. A recent survey of 1,817 general practitioners in England found that the mean job stressor scores were significantly higher in the 1990 and 1993 samples than were the scores for comparable samples of physicians polled in 1987.[6] And the Canadian Medical Association's 1998 national survey of more than 3,500 physicians was summarized in this way:

> "Canada's physicians appear to be a stressed-out, fed-up and cranky lot as the close of the century approaches. . . . Never have so many physicians worked so much for so little income and so little gratitude."[1 (p. 525)]

To truly understand physician job stress and career satisfaction, we must expand our thinking. Certainly, excessive work can contribute to burnout. But this may be due more to what excessive working precludes (eg, time spent relaxing, enjoying family relationships and avocational interests, etc) than to any direct effect of long work hours. Remember: Stress that is highly demanding but also meaningful and controllable is healthy stress, not the sort that promotes burnout.[28] Our counseling and consulting experiences suggest that what *really* stresses today's physicians is feeling betrayed, or double-crossed.

PSYCHOLOGICAL "CONTRACTS" AND THE COSTS OF FEELING DOUBLE-CROSSED

It has been argued that the ongoing restructuring of the health care industry has largely ignored human and organizational elements.[9] When this happens, the psychological "contracts" that were stated or implied in a physician's relationships with patients, colleagues, and organizations are violated.

A psychological contract has to do with expectations about what one will receive in return for one's efforts. Schaufeli explained that the psychological contract for physicians involves many things, including the expectation of a reasonable workload; support from the organization; esteem, autonomy, and dignity at work; supportive, fair dealings with colleagues; and appropriate degrees of patient collaboration and appreciation for the physician's efforts.[29] When psychological contracts are violated, the sense of having been double-crossed results. As defined by Webster,[30] to double cross is "to cheat or betray an associate."

The aforementioned national survey of Canadian physicians yielded a telling quotation from one physician who was clearly suffering the pain of the double cross.

> "I believe that most physicians unconsciously contracted with society to pursue their profession to the utmost of their ability and energy, to keep up their skills and do whatever was needed to promote patient care. In return, we expected respect, the equipment to do the job and freedom from financial anxieties. All 3 of these expectations have been abrogated, yet we continue to fulfill our side of the contract in confusion, disbelief and a sense of betrayal."[1 (p. 528)]

A physician who feels double-crossed is at risk of losing trust and of reneging on commitments to his or her organization or to the relationships that perpetuated the double cross. One result is increased stress and diminished morale, not only for physicians but for those who turn to them for leadership—their patients, hospital staff, and office personnel.[31]

If we are accurate in our hypothesis that a physician who feels double-crossed suffers relationship tensions, it is reasonable to say that a double-crossed physician is at risk of burnout. This is because convincing research[32] suggests that relationship stress may have more deleterious consequences on health than work stress. Harmonious relationships, on the other hand, have been found to enhance stress resilience.[33] It therefore behooves us to discuss the double-cross phenomena, which may affect a physician's interpersonal life, both at work and at home. We have identified five major sources of double cross: loss of autonomy; changes in the patient–physician relationship; work–family conflicts; conflicts with peers, staff, and administrators; and lack of collegiality, particularly in the wake of having made a mistake.

High-Demand/Low-Control Stress: Loss of Autonomy

The intrusion of business agendas into the medical workplace has resulted in the most frequently cited cause for physician disillusionment: loss of autonomy.[27]

Example:

> Karen, a pediatrician whose practice was recently bought by a large health maintenance organization (HMO), expressed her dismay in these words: "I thought that this was going to be a good deal. I expected regular hours and no business worries. In fact, it's turned into a nightmare. I now work twice as hard to make significantly less money, all the while having to endure the worst administrative headaches imaginable. It seems like overnight, I went from being an autonomous professional to a member of a corporation I don't even like!"

As mentioned in our introductory comments, Karasek and colleagues documented the toxic health effects that come from work that is highly demanding but that leaves workers with low "decision latitude" or control. Specifically, high-demand/low-control work stress has been found to correlate with elevated rates of coronary heart disease and death.[34] And in a study of nearly 300 American hospital employees, levels of burnout, psychosomatic symptoms, depression, and job dissatisfaction were significantly higher in situations characterized by high job demands and low control.[35]

But this same research lends some hope to physicians. For example, researchers have shown that work stress is more affected by the inability to control the pace of one's work than by the actual level of one's workload and that perceptions are powerful determinants of outcomes. In a Swedish study,[36] it was shown that even the illusion of control lowered levels of harmful urinary catecholamines in Swedish assembly-line workers when compared to those who worked at the same pace but believed they had no control over pace. Our consulting experiences suggest that physicians are better able to manage stress when: (1) they are offered hope that their problems are solvable and (2) they are taught specific skills and concepts that enhance their abilities to manage their relationships. In short, when they are helped to increase their sense of control, physicians cope better. For this reason, among others, a physician who is facing an unwanted swirl of workplace changes would be well advised to become involved in some way with the administrative processes that are driving the changes. Even if doing so does not result in actual control of the process, it may, at minimum, increase the *perception* of control and thereby diminish the toxicity of the change.

A final important note: Research in this area has shown that when lack of social support is added to the high-demand/low-control paradigm, the toxic effect is amplified. Specifically, "isolated high-strain" jobs[37]—those characterized by high demands, low control, and low support—have been found to predict both psychological health complaints[38,39] and somatic symptoms.[40] This fact underscores the importance of moving beyond the relationship-damaging consequences of the double-cross phenomena.

Changes in the Patient–Physician Relationship

Changes in the patient–physician relationship constitute another source of double cross. The news media is quick to point out the various ways that patients may suffer when physicians are forced by managed care to limit the time they spend with each individual. What has not been so publicized is the effect this process has on physician well-being. The loss of positive feedback from patients, which comes with the "hurried-physician" mode of medical practice, creates a dangerous lack of reciprocity in the psychological balance of the patient–physician relationship.[17] As mentioned earlier, physicians need and value certain rewards such as patient gratitude, improvement, or an effort to get well in return for their efforts.[17] If these rewards disappear, physicians may grow to feel that they put more effort into the relationships with their patients than they receive in return. Lack of reciprocity may then drain the physician's emotional resources, leading to emotional exhaustion.[41]

Example:

> In the 23 years we have known Adam, we have seen him progress from an idealistic resident invested in pleasing others to a hurried, overstressed, middle-aged physician whose brusque manner often leaves his patients questioning whether or not he even listens to them. When he came to us for counseling mandated by the risk management committee in his multispecialty group practice, he lamented: "I'm here because my patients are complaining that I don't show enough ´caring` for them. What a joke! I've spent my life caring: I've cared enough to work the hours I've worked; I've cared enough to save so many of their lives; and I've cared enough to keep showing up, even though I know that half of them don't even follow the advice I give them. *I'm* the one who feels uncared for. I'm tired of ungrateful, uncooperative patients who expect doctors to be all things to them, regardless of whether or not *they* hold up *their* end of the bargain."

Work–Family Conflicts

Regardless of gender, stage of career, or marital status, a major stressor cited by physicians today is work–family conflict.[42] In *The Medical Marriage,* we extensively addressed the family dynamics that stem from work–family conflicts experienced by physicians and their loved ones.[43] In Chapter 5, we outline recommendations for managing this process. Here, we emphasize an important point drawn from research in the medical workplace: family-responsive work environments and supportive supervisors and colleagues have been shown to reduce felt-strain for physicians and other medical professionals.[44-46] On the other hand, double cross results when medical administrators ignore work–family issues, physicians ignore or complicate each other's work–family dilemmas, or a physician's family fails to support the physician's role-juggling efforts.

Examples:

> Marie, a female physician: "When I took maternity leave during my residency, I rather expected to encounter stated or implied criticism from some of the attendings. What I never expected was the "cold shoulder" I got from my fellow residents. And my female colleagues were the most critical! They acted as though my choosing to get pregnant was a setback to the cause of women in medicine."

Luka, a male physician: "I've been a partner in this practice for nearly 9 years. For 9 years, I've worked side-by-side with this group. I know that I've done my part; maybe even more than my fair share. I've been reasonable. I've been a team player. So I just can't understand this: None of my partners would agree to cover for me when my mother was hospitalized last month. Not one. This makes me wonder what kind of people they are."

Thomas, a male physician: "I know that my wife met with you last week to complain about what an uninvolved husband and father I am. Well, let me say a few things about the other side of the coin. First, I spend more hands-on time with my kids and with my wife than any man in the history of my family ever has. My father was *never* around. And my mother never complained. Secondly, I guarantee you that I'm home more than any of my colleagues are. In fact, my partners at work are busting my chops because they want me to be like them: On any given day, they'd much rather be in the hospital than at home. I'm having my commitment to work questioned because I *do* make it my business to get home at a reasonable hour. I'm tired of this. I'm getting criticized from both ends."

Conflicts with Peers, Staff, and Administrators

According to a "flashmail survey" responded to by 115 members of the American Academy of Physician Executives in 1999,[47] conflict with the people they supervise, work with, and report to ranks highest on the list of causes of stress for physicians. The areas of conflict noted in the survey are summarized following:

Peer Conflict

Schedules and calendars
Approaches to patient management
Sharing workload
Clinic or laboratory space
Management of budget for a group/unit
Balancing patient care, teaching, and research
Authorship disputes
Failure to deal with their low performers

Conflict with People Physicians Supervise

Conflict among supervisees that compromises work
Expectations for performance
Dealing with the low performer

Workloads and schedules
Inappropriate personal relationships at work
Volume and quality of work
Interactions with supervisor
Unwillingness to change practice or behavior
Supervision outside the hierarchy

Conflict with Authority Figures

Disagreement about values
Lack of consistency in their actions
Micromanagement
Unfair treatment
Discrimination
Salary negotiations
Broken promises
Clinical and other workload
Ethical dilemmas

Of course, the results from this very small, informal survey cannot be generalized to all physicians. But even this small survey suggests that the quality of work relationships may affect a physician's well-being. Our consulting experiences suggest that double cross in the medical workplace comes in many forms. A few examples follow.

Examples:

Practice X, a large, multispecialty medical practice, asked for our consultation to help deal with intragroup, interpersonal conflicts that were paralyzing their operations. A festering problem concerned allegations of racism within the group. Indeed, the practice was culturally diverse. It consisted of seven Caucasians, three African Americans, two Hindus, one Peruvian, two Indians, and one Mexican American. Unfortunately, the busy physicians in this group had never taken the time to learn about each of the cultures represented. They simply kept working hard at their grueling clinical schedules and ignored the escalating tensions and diminishing morale within the group. By the time of our intervention, accumulated hurt feelings and resentments were threatening the very future of the organization.

Practice Y, a group of seven surgeons, operated on the border of chaos most of the time. Even though their "lump and split" model of pay resulted in equal pay for every surgeon, allegations of professional sabotage ran rampant within the group. Certain physicians were notorious for disparaging their partners in front of valued referral sources, hoarding cases rather than evenly distributing the work-load, and ostracizing certain of their partners.

Practice Z agreed to settle for deeply discounted reimbursement fees in order to join the provider panel of an HMO that was owned by their county hospital. When Practice Z discovered that their referrals and clinical services accounted for more than 60% of the hospital's gross revenues, they asked for what seemed to them to be reasonable and fair concessions. These included requests that the hospital provide them with a sleeping room to accommodate on-call physicians, provide adequate nursing staff to facilitate their massive volume of patient flow, and create medical directorships for various of their partners as a legal means of reimbursing them for the many hours of continuing education they provided to the hospital's nursing staff. The hospital administration denied all of the physicians' requests, stating the concern that, if they granted the physicians their wishes, the hospital might be perceived to be giving financial "kickbacks" to these preferred referral sources.

Fear of Mistakes and Lack of Collegiality

Through all stages of a medical career, physician well-being may be negatively affected by fear of making mistakes and by lack of peer support when a mistake is made. Leape[48] put it this way:

". . . physicians, not unlike test pilots, come to view an error as a failure of character—you weren't careful, you didn't try hard enough. This kind of thinking lies behind a common reaction by clinicians: 'How can there be an error without negligence?'"

Such fears are especially prevalent during medical training. Mizrahi[49] asked young interns: "What were your most memorable experiences during training?" Twenty-one percent of the replies concerned actual or potential mistakes, and serious and even fatal mistakes were reported by 50% of the new interns interviewed in the first 2 months of their jobs. Firth-Cozens and colleagues surveyed medical residents and found that their main stressors did not include long work hours; the main stressors were making mistakes, dealing with death and dying, and *their relationships with senior physicians*.[50,51] Stress levels of physicians-in-training are especially likely to escalate when they do not receive adequate feedback or are subjected to poor educational supervision.[50,52]

Example:

Marital problems brought Joseph to our offices, but unresolved posttraumatic stress syndrome related to his residency was his real problem. Within three sessions, Joseph began to recount the grueling schedule his neurosurgery training necessitated and the often brutal way he was treated by senior residents and attendings. "I've always had a secret fear that I was an 'impostor;' not really as smart and competent as others think I am. The senior resident during my second year seemed to know this, and he played on it. He would even tease me about it in front of the other residents. Every time a bad outcome happened—even if I wasn't involved—he'd sarcastically ask if I was the one who had "killed" the patient.

And he wasn't the only one. I accepted this residency to train with Dr (X). I couldn't believe it when, during my first month there, he asked me, "How did you ever get here? What *ever* gave you the notion that you could be a neurosurgeon?"

Maybe that was just his way of getting my attention. I don't know. But I do know that I never stopped being afraid of him. Not in 5 years. I've been miserable for 5 years."

Lack of collegiality is not just a young person's issue. Conflicts that stem from generational differences among medical partners can also result in double-cross phenomena. For example, aging physicians may feel double-crossed by younger partners who fail to facilitate their late-career exit strategies.

Example:

Bill, a physician: "I truly cannot believe this. I started this practice. I recruited and hired every one of the nine partners in this group. Now *they* are trying to tell *me* that I can't slow down and remain a voting partner in my own practice! I'm willing to sacrifice income for dropping out of the on-call rotation. That ought to be enough. They act as though I'm asking for something that I don't deserve. What they don't see is that they are refusing me something that should have been part of the deal that comes with working as hard as I have for all these years."

Finally, as will be shown later, the distressing effects of lack of peer support are especially poignant if a physician faces the ultimate double cross—a medical malpractice suite.

Postlitigation Syndrome: The Special Stress
Approximately one third of physicians are eventually subjected to a medical malpractice suit.[53] Being sued can seriously damage a physician's well-being and taint his or her overall attitudes and

feelings about practicing medicine. In a controlled study of 171 sued physicians and 100 nonsued physicians, the sued physicians stated that they found the practice of medicine to be significantly less rewarding and satisfying after legal action.[7]

The pain of a malpractice suit is significantly compounded when medical colleagues fail to offer open support to the accused and their families. A recent survey of more than 100 British physicians documented the importance of support from friends, colleagues, management, and outside professionals,[54] especially during times of stress. And in a study of family physicians,[55] almost all of those surveyed stated a need for support after making a serious medical error. But, unfortunately, only one-third stated that they would be willing to provide support unconditionally to colleagues.[55] Silence or tacit or blatant blame from one's peers is the opposite of what these families most need in order to cope well.

Example:

> Theresa, a physician: "I haven't received one call from any of my colleagues since the article appeared in the paper telling all the gory details of this malpractice suit. Not one. This nightmare has been going on for 18 months, and I feel totally isolated. I find myself avoiding the doctors' lounge at the hospital. I've got no one to talk to about this. My husband is tired of the topic, and I'm terrified."

These five factors (loss of autonomy; changes in the patient–physician relationship; work–family conflicts; conflicts with peers, staff, and administrators; and lack of collegiality, particularly in the wake of having made a mistake) can combine to leave a physician feeling double-crossed and traumatized. In the broadest sense, ". . . traumatic events (are) those that shatter peoples' beliefs that they live in a meaningful, predictable world."[56] According to Epstein,[57] trauma can damage us on four levels: our beliefs about the benignity of the world, the possibility of justice, the trustworthiness of other people, and our self-worth.

Physicians who have been traumatized in these ways tend to settle into obsessive rumination regarding their plight. Free-floating anxiety may result and lead to agitation, irritability, and/or depression. As will be seen later, effectively managing such pain hinges on creating safer and more nurturing life arenas.

TOWARD EFFECTIVE EMOTIONAL MANAGEMENT

Even if the health care environment does not become a more physician-friendly place (and we hope that it does!), physicians can help protect themselves and each other from untoward stress effects. Doing so requires making the medical workplace a supportive, positive, interpersonal culture, one that buffers, rather than compounds, the effects of double cross. This effort requires that individual physicians commit to learning EEM skills.

Effective emotional management hinges on making the right choices to shape the "territory" of one's life.[43,58,59] Fundamentally, we propose that well-being is shaped by choices that fall into three categories: *How* we manage our physical, emotional, cognitive, psychological, and spiritual needs; *whom* we affiliate with; and *where* we spend our time. Further, we propose that it is difficult to remain healthy and happy if you live or work in a toxic "territory" created by nonnurturing choices in any of these three areas. The remainder of this book offers practical guidelines for understanding and shaping different components of your life territory. We close this chapter with five recommendations that are components of EEM and are effective ways to prevent and remediate the double-cross phenomena outlined earlier.

Manage Your Attitude

It is important to be realistic about work today.[60] In medicine, as in other industries, new paradigms have been and will continue to be created. Ongoing cost-cutting efforts will mean that success requires physicians to blend business savvy and creative problem solving into their armamentarium of professional skills. Greater demands, coupled with fewer people employed on-site to do the work, will likely mean that physicians can expect increased work pressures. It is also likely that the need to integrate information technology into the delivery of patient care will grow.

This does not mean that you have to revel in unwanted changes. But there are attitudinal lessons to be learned from researchers like Salvatore Maddi and Suzanne Kobasa Ouellette, who popularized the term *psychological hardiness*.[61] In their 8-year study of what differentiates executives likely to get sick from those who stayed well after the AT&T divestiture, they found that three attitudinal qualities increased the odds 7-fold that the executives would stay healthy:

- Challenge: Stress-hardy people learn to see what faces them as a personal, career, and organizational opportunity rather than as a disaster.
- Control: The stress-hardy learn to believe that they have the power to make things come out all right in the end, both for themselves and for their organization and profession.
- Commitment: Stress-hardy individuals also maintain strong bonds and emotional ties to their organization, profession, family, and community.

Make Self-Protective Choices When Possible

Aldwin[62] observed that individuals are put at risk when their subculture involves values or standards that lead to behaviors that foster toxic stress, rather than stress resilience. For this reason, it is a mistake for any physician to ignore the interpersonal "culture" of his work and home environments. Rather, physicians should accept that healthy coping necessitates making self-protective choices or corrections in work and family relationships.

Hospitals and medical practices differ greatly in the levels of stress experienced by their medical staff. For example, research has suggested that, in general, staff members in larger hospitals tend to report poorer scores on measures of mental health than do their colleagues working in smaller hospitals.[63] Furthermore, our consulting experiences suggest that individual medical practices vary greatly along the continuum of nurturing versus toxic interpersonal dynamics.

We have been amazed at how often we hear physicians who are locked into toxic conflict with colleagues say that, from the outset of the partnership, it was clear that interpersonal tensions existed; but this information was ignored or devalued in the process of making the decision to take the job. Physicians would be well-advised to value the variable of personal style and preference when considering career placements. Ignoring such information or intuition when choosing a professional partnership sets the stage for later, costly conflicts.

Learn to Be a Team-Builder

As was mentioned earlier, in the general health psychology literature, social support has been shown to attenuate the negative
health effects of high-demand/low-control stress.[64,65] A specific
form of social support comes when you work in a cohesive team.
To succeed in the new millennium, physicians must take the lead
in creating collaborative work teams.[66] Paternalistic or authoritarian styles of managing others or delivering medical care are generally ineffective in today's medical workplace. They must be
replaced with management and clinical styles that promote collaboration between physicians, allied health professionals,
patients, and families.

It is also imperative that physicians who work together commit themselves to maintaining collegiality. At minimum, this
might involve participating in local, state, and national medical
organizations. For physicians who practice together, collegiality
requires regular participation in team-building activities by all
members of the medical group. Too often, medical groups skip
this crucial aspect of organizational development. At no time are
the costs of this error of omission more apparent than when multiple, independent medical practices merge into large, complex
medical corporations. Busy physicians—especially those who feel
double-crossed by the need to merge into larger groups—find it
easy to justify absenting themselves from the various meetings,
group affairs, or corporate retreats that are typically necessary in
order to develop or maintain a sense of teamwork.

Resources for developing the interpersonal skills necessary for
team-building are available in the literature.[43,66–69] We devote
Section II of this book to extensive discussion of various communication and negotiation skills required to promote teamwork. In
Chapter 13, we outline our thoughts on team-building.

Be Honest About the Risks and Symptoms of Burnout

Medical training teaches physicians to ignore their own symptoms of distress. This is a dangerous form of denial that can lead
to both personal and relationship problems. The evolving medical
workplace should flag physicians at risk of burnout and offer
prophylactic or corrective interventions to them. Be particularly

concerned by indications of extreme perfectionism early in one's career. Firth-Cozens[70] demonstrated that medical students and residents who were highly self-critical tended to manifest high levels of late-career stress and to experience difficulties in their relationships with senior colleagues. All physicians, but especially novice physicians who evidence high self-criticism, would benefit from medical education and mentoring that emphasizes the ubiquity of medical errors and teaches strategies for coping with them.[70] The goal is to shape realistic attitudes and constructive approaches for dealing with what otherwise may become perfectionistic expectations that will compromise well-being and complicate interpersonal dynamics.

Offer Prophylactic Training in Effective Emotional Management Skills

Any medical organization would be wise to make readily available to its members training in life skills such as conflict management, work–family balancing strategies, and overall *EEM* skills. Research supports this claim. For example, numerous studies[71-74] have shown that multifaceted stress management training can help physicians cope more effectively with work-related stressors. Mushin and colleagues[71] demonstrated the efficacy of a 12-session psychoeducational/support program for residents that addressed such issues as time management, interaction with nurses, dealing with difficult people, and family concerns. The St. Paul Fire and Marine Insurance Company project found that a multicomponent stress intervention with physicians even reduced medication errors by as much as 50%.[75] And a recent survey of 882 physicians in the United Kingdom[76] found that having good relationships with patients, relatives, and staff was protective against burnout. Feeling insufficiently trained in communication and management skills, however, correlated with increased risk of burnout. Further, of the physicians polled in this UK study, only 45% judged that they had received adequate training in communication skills and only 22% in management skills.

In addition to improving a physician's quality of life, training in the skills needed to respond to others with sensitivity and compassion decreases the occurrence of formal complaints and acts of malpractice litigation.[77] It has been shown that, often, a malpractice suit is preceded by difficulties in the patient–physician relationship.[78]

Recent studies showed that what distinguished obstetric and gynecology specialists with high levels of malpractice claims from colleagues who had low levels of malpractice suites was not the quality of their care; it was differences in attitudes, sensitivity levels,
and communication skills.[79,80]

CONCLUSIONS

Some[47,66] have proposed that traditional medical training predisposes physicians to cope in ways that are maladaptive in today's
world. Historically, the medical workplace functioned as an exception to the business and administrative rules of other industries.
This fact, coupled with the lofty position of power and authority
that was assigned to physicians by our culture, generally allowed
them to avoid areas outside their realm of competency. In addition
to facing more complicated medical challenges than any prior generation, the average physician today is faced with the complex
dynamics occurring in corporate boardrooms. They must learn to
hold their own when dealing with a new breed of patients who do
not defer to them as all-knowing authorities, but who, instead,
demand relationships, collaboration, and sharing of power. And
the need to share authority with medical administrators and teams
of allied health professionals is unprecedented. In addition, physicians today, like most busy professionals, must negotiate their way
through the complex maze created by the multiple roles that define
the contemporary family.[43,81] They must learn to juggle busy careers,
hands-on participation in family life, and appropriate self-care.

These demands of a twenty-first century life in medicine
require many physicians to reconsider their socialization, training,
experience, and psychology.[47] Indeed, "…the age of the command-
ing general and the obedient, dependent, and loyal soldier is
passing."[82 (p. 55)] How physicians deal emotionally with the changed
paradigms they live and work in sets the tone that determines
quality of life for themselves and others. Anger management
expert Henrie Weisinger put it this way:

"Emotions can no longer be thought of as insignificant factors or out of
place when it comes to doing business. Quite the contrary: Emotions can be
powerful tools that strongly influence productivity and improve our interpersonal
effectiveness."[83 (p. 54)]

Clearly, the need for physicians to learn and practice EEM skills has never been greater. For many physicians, doing so requires a revamping of self-care strategies. We turn to this important topic in our next chapter.

CHAPTER 1—REFERENCES

1. Sullivan P, Buske L. Results from CMA's huge 1998 physician survey point to a dispirited profession. *Can Med Assoc J.* 1998;159:525–528.

2. Hadley J, Cantor JC, Wilke RJ, Feeder J, Cohen AB. Young physicians most and least likely to have second thoughts about career in medicine. *Acad Med.* 1992;67:180–190.

3. Harvey LK, Shubat SC. *Physician Opinion on Health Care Issues.* Issues and Communications Research. Chicago, Ill: American Medical Association; April 1989 and April 1990.

4. Skolnik NS, Smith DR, Diamond J. Professional satisfaction and dissatisfaction of family physicians. *J Fam Pract.* 1993;37:257–263.

5. Chan WS, Sunshine JH, Owen JB, Shaffer KA. U.S. radiologists' satisfaction in their profession. *Radiology.* 1995;194:649–656.

6. Howie J, Porter M. Stress and interventions for stress in general practitioners. In: Firth-Cozens J, Payne R, eds. *Stress in Health Professionals: Psychological and Organisational Causes and Interventions.* New York, NY: John Wiley & Sons; 1999:163–176.

7. Cooper CL, Rout U, Fargher B. Mental health, job satisfaction, and job stress among general practitioners. *BMJ.* 1989;298:366–370.

8. Firth-Cozens J. The psychological problems of doctors. In: Firth-Cozens J, Payne R, eds. *Stress in Health Professionals: Psychological and Organisational Causes and Interventions.* New York, NY: John Wiley & Sons; 1999:79–91.

9. Murphy LR. Organisational interventions to reduce stress in health care professionals. In: Firth-Cozens J, Payne R, eds. *Stress in Health Professionals: Psychological and Organisational Causes and Interventions.* New York, NY: John Wiley & Sons; 1999:149–162.

10. Lin LS, Yager J, Cope D, Leake B. Health status, job satisfaction, job stress, and life satisfaction among academic and clinical faculty. *JAMA.* 1985;254:2775–2782.

11. DiMatteo MR, Sherbourne CD, Hays RD, Ordway L, Dravitz RL, McGlynn EA, Kaplan S, Rogers WH. Physicians' characteristics influence patients' adherence to medical treatment: Results from the Medical Outcomes Study. *Health Psychol.* 1993;12:93–102.

12. Lazarus RS. The trivialization of distress. In: Rosen JC, Solomon LJ, eds. *Prevention in Health Psychology.* Hanover, NH: University Press of New England; 1985:279–298.

13. Maslach C. *Burnout: The Cost of Caring.* Englewood Cliffs, NJ: Prentice-Hall; 1982.

14. Maslach C, Jackson SE, Leiter MP. *Maslach Burnout Inventory Manual.* 3rd ed. Palo Alto, Calif: Consulting Psychologists Press, Inc; 1996.

15. Schaufeli WB, Enzmann D. *The Burnout Companion to Study and Practice: A Critical Analysis.* London: Taylor & Francis; 1998.

16. Gross EB. Gender differences in physician stress. *JAMWA.* 1992;47:107–114.

17. Schaufeli W. Burnout. In: Firth-Cozens J, Payne R, eds. *Stress in Health Professionals: Psychological and Organisational Causes and Interventions.* New York, NY: John Wiley & Sons; 1999:17–32

18. McCranie EW, Brandsma JM. Personality antecedents of burnout among middle-aged physicians. *Behav Med.* 1988(Spring):30–36.

19. McCrae RR, Costa PT. Personality, coping, and coping effectiveness in an adult sample. *J Pers.* 1986;54:385–405.

20. Krakowski AJ. Stress and the practice of medicine: The myth and the reality. *J of Psychosom Res.* 1982;26:91–98.

21. Mawardi BH. Satisfactions, dissatisfactions and causes of stress in medical practice. *JAMA.* 1979;241:1483–1486.

22. Clarke TA, Maniscalco WM, Taylor-Brown S, et al. Job satisfaction and stress among neonatologists. *Pediatrics.* 1984;74:52–57.

23. Anwar RAH. A longitudinal study of residency-trained emergency physicians. *Ann Emerg Med.* 1983;12:20/21–24/55.

24. McCranie EW, Hornsby JL, Calvert JC. Practice and career satisfaction among residency trained family physicians: A national survey. *J Fam Pract.* 1982;14:1107–1114.

25. Linn LS, Kosecoff J, Clark V, et al. *Preliminary Evaluation Report: Provider Survey Data.* Los Angeles, CA: Robert Wood Johnson Teaching Hospital General Medicine Group Practice Program; 1982.

26. Simpson LA, Grant L. Sources and magnitude of job stress among physicians. *J Behav Med.* 1991;14:27–42.

27. Chuck JM, Nesbitt TS, Kwan J, Kam SM. Is being a doctor still fun? *West J Med.* 1993;159:665–669.

28. Csikszentmihalyi M. *Flow: The Psychology of Optimal Experience.* New York, NY: Harper Perennial; 1990.

29. Schaufeli WB, Van Dierendonck D, Van Gorp K. Burnout and reciprocity: Towards a dual-level social exchange model. *Work and Stress.* 1996;3:225–237.

30. *The New Lexicon Webster's Dictionary of the English Language.* New York, NY: Lexicon Publications, Inc.; 1989:280.

31. President's Advisory Commission. *Quality First: Better Health Care for all Americans.* Washington, DC: Advisory Commission on Consumer Protection and Quality in the Health Care Industry; 1998.

32. Coyne JC, DeLongis A. Going beyond social support: The role of social relationships in adaptation. *J Consult Clin Psychol.* 1986;54:454–460.

33. Spendlove DC, Reed BD, Whitman N, Slattery ML, French TK, Horwood, K. Marital adjustment among house staff and new attorneys. *Acad Med.* 1990;65:599–603.

34. Karasek RA, Theorell T, Schwartz JE, Schnall PL, Pieper CF, Michela JL. Job characteristics in relation to the prevalence of myocardial infarction in the US health examination survey (HES) and the health and nutrition examination survey (HANES). 1988. *Am J Public Health.* 78:910–918.

35. Landsbergis PA. Occupational stress among health care workers: A test of the job demands-control model. *J of Organ Behav.* 1988;9:217–239.

36. Frankenhauser M. Psychobiological aspects of life stress. In: Levine S, Ursin H, eds. *Coping and Health.* New York, NY: Plenum; 1980:203–223.

37. Geurts S, Rutte C, Peeters M. Antecedents and consequences of work-home interference among medical residents. *Soc Sci Med.* 1999;48:1135–1148.

38. Karasek RA, Theorell T. *Healthy Work: Stress, Productivity and the Reconstruction of Working Life.* New York, NY: Basic Books; 1990.

39. Johnson JV, Hall EM. Social support in the work environment and cardiovascular disease: A cross-sectional study of a random sample of the Swedish working population. *Am J Public Health.* 1994;78:1336–1342.

40. Parkes KR, Mendham CA, vonRabenau C. Social support and the demand-discretion model of job stress: Tests and additive and interactive effects in two samples. *J Vocational Behav.* 1994;44:91–113.

41. Buunk BP, Schaufeli WB. Burnout: A perspective from social comparison theory. In: Schaufeli WB, Maslach C, Marek T, eds. *Professional Burnout: Recent Developments in Theory and Research.* Washington, DC: Taylor & Francis; 1993:53–69.

42. Graham J, Ramirez AJ, Cull A, Finlay I, Hoy A, Richards MA. Job stress and satisfaction among palliative physicians. *Palliat Med.* 1996;10:185–194.

43. Sotile WM, Sotile MO. *The Medical Marriage: Sustaining Healthy Relationships for Physicians and Their Families.* Chicago, Ill: American Medical Association; 2000.

44. Ducker D. Research on women physicians with multiple roles: A feminist perspective. *JAMWA.* 1994;49:78–84.

45. Greenberger E, Goldberg W, Hamil S, et al. Contributions of a supportive work environment to parents' well-being and orientation to work. *Am J Community Psychol.* 1989;17:755–783.

46. Repetti RL. Individual and common components of the social environment at work and psychological well-being. *J Pers Soc Psychol.* 1987;52:710–720.

47. Aschenbrener CA, Siders CT. Managing low-to-mid intensity conflict in the health care setting. *The Physician Executive.* 1999;25:44–50.

48. Leape LL. Error in medicine. *JAMA.* 1994;272:1851–1857.

49. Mizrahi T. Managing medical mistakes: Ideology, insularity and accountability among internists in training. *Soc Sci Med.* 1984;19:135–145.

50. Firth-Cozens J. Emotional distress in junior house officers. *BMJ.* 1987;295:533–536.

51. Richardson C. Shadowing: The Leicester experience. In: Paice E, ed. *Delivering the New Doctor.* Edinburgh: ASME; 1998.

52. Moss F, Paice E. Getting things right for the doctor in training. Firth-Cozens J, Payne R, eds. *Stress in Health Professionals: Psychological and Organisational Causes and Interventions.* New York, NY: John Wiley & Sons; 1999:203–218.

53. Gonzalez ML. *Medical Professional Liability Trends, 1985–1997.* Chicago, Ill: American Medical Association Center for Health Policy Research; 1999.

54. Bark P, Vincent C, Oliveri L, Jones A. Impact of litigation on senior clinicians: Implications for risk management. *Quality in Health Care.* 1997;6:7–13.

55. Newman MC. The emotional impact of mistakes on family physicians. *Arch Fam Med.* 1996;5:71–75.

56. Benner P, Roskies E, Lazarus RS. Stress and coping under extreme circumstances. In: Dimsdale JE, ed. *Survivors, Victims, and Perpetrators: Essays on the Nazi Holocaust.* Washington, DC: Hemisphere; 1980:219–258.

57. Epstein S. The self-concept, the traumatic neurosis, and the structure of personality. In: Ozer D, Healy JH, Stewart AJ, eds. *Perspectives in Personality, Vol. 3.* London: Kingsley; 1991:63–98.

58. Sotile WM, Sotile MO. Conflict management, part 1: How to shape positive relationships in medical practices and hospitals. *The Physician Executive.* 1999;25:57–61.

59. Sotile WM, Sotile MO. Conflict management, part 2: How to shape positive relationships in medical practices and hospitals. *The Physician Executive.* 1999;25:51–55.

60. Reinhold BB. *Toxic Work.* New York, NY: Dutton; 1996.

61. Maddi S, Kobasa S. *The Hardy Executive: Health Under Stress.* Chicago, Ill: Dorsey Professional Books, Dow-Jones-Irvin; 1984.

62. Aldwin C. Does age affect the stress and coping process? Implications of age differences in perceived control. *J Gerontol.* 1991;46:174–180.

63. Wall TD, Bolden RI, Borril CS, Carter AJ, Golya DA, Hardy GE, Haynes CE, Rick JE, Sahpiro D, West M. Minor psychiatric disorder in NHS trust staff: Occupational and gender differences. *Br J of Psychiatry.* 1997;171:519–523.

64. Luecken LJ, et al. Stress in employed women: Impact of marital status and children at home on neurohormone output and home strain. *Psychosom Med.* 1990;52:42–58.

65. Williams R. Stress management training boosts social support in married working mothers. Paper presented at the Fourth International Congress of Behavioral Medicine. Washington, DC, March, 1996.

66. Marcus LJ. *Renegotiating Health Care: Resolving Conflict to Build Collaboration.* San Francisco, CA: Jossey-Bass Publishers; 1995.

67. Ryan KD, Oestreich DK. *Driving Fear out of the Workplace,* 2nd ed. San Francisco, Calif: Jossey-Bass Publishers; 1998.

68. Fisher R, Ury W. *Getting to Yes: Negotiating Agreement Without Giving In,* 2nd ed. New York, NY: Penguin Books; 1991.

69. Goldman LS, Myers M, Dickstein LJ. *The Handbook of Physician Health: The Essential Guide to Understanding the Health Care Needs of Physicians.* Chicago, Ill: American Medical Association; 2000.

70. Firth-Cozens J. Depression in doctors. In: Katona C, Robertson MM, eds. *Depression and Physical Illness.* Chichester: Wiley; 1997.

71. Mushin IC, Matteson MT, Lynch EC. Developing a resident assistance program: Beyond the support group model. *Arch Intern Med.* 1993;153:729–733.

72. Rowe MM. Teaching health-care providers coping: Results of a two-year study. *J Behav Med.* 1999;22:511–527.

73. Hooley I. Circumventing burnout in AIDS care. *Am J Occup Ther*. 1997;51:759–766.

74. Schaubroeck J, Merritt DE. Divergent effects of job control on coping with work stressors: The key role of self-efficacy. *Acad Manage J*. 1997;40:738–754.

75. Jones JW, Barge BN, Steffy BD, Fay LM, Kuntz LK, Wuebeker LJ. Stress and medical malpractice: Organizational risk assessment and intervention. *J Appl Psychol*. 1988;73:727–735.

76. Ramirez AJ, Graham J, Richards MA, Cull A, Gregory WM. Mental health of hospital consultants: The effects of stress and satisfaction at work. *Lancet*. 1996;347:724–728.

77. Vincent C, Young M, Phillips A. Why do people sue doctors? A study of patients and relatives taking legal action. *Lancet*. 1994;343:1609–1613.

78. Shapiro RS, Simpson DE, Lawrence SL, Talsky AM, Sobocinski KA, Schiedermayer DL. A survey of sued and non-sued physicians and suing patients. *Arch Intern Med*. 1989;149:2190–2196.

79. Entman SS, Glass CA, Hickson GB, Githens PB, Whetten-Goldstein K, Sloan FA. The relationship between malpractice claims history and subsequent obstetric care. *JAMA*. 1994;272:1588–1591.

80. Hickson GB, Clayton EW, Entman SS, Miller CS, Githens PB, Whetten-Goldstein K, Sloan FA. Obstetricians' prior malpractice experience and patients' satisfaction with care. *JAMA*. 1994;272:1583–1587.

81. Sotile WM, Sotile MO. *Beat Stress Together: The BEST Way to a Passionate Marriage, a Healthy Family, and a Productive Life*. New York, NY: John Wiley & Sons; 1999.

82. Kilburg RR. *Executive Coaching: Developing Managerial Wisdom in a World of Chaos*. Washington, DC: American Psychological Association; 2000.

83. Weisinger H. *Anger at Work: Learning the Art of Anger Management on the Job*. New York, NY: William Morrow & Co; 1995.

Self-Assessment: How Are You Doing?

"You can't expect your patients to feel any better than you do."

Wayne and Mary Sotile

Do physicians practice what they preach? Answers to this question vary widely. A recent book on physician well-being published by the American Medical Association[1] asserted that physicians generally live reasonably healthy personal lives. For example, less than 4% of the physician population smoke cigarettes, as compared to 25% of the general population.

Many researchers, however, have raised serious concerns about various aspects of physician health. Heim[2] summarized research conducted with Finnish, Danish, British, Japanese, and American physician cohorts and concluded that the overall mortality rate for physicians is higher than that of all other professionals combined. Specifically, compared to controls, physicians have increased incidences of depression, strokes, and cardiovascular disease.

The life span of physicians is shorter than that of socioeconomically comparable groups,[3] and female physicians, specifically, have been found to have a 10-year lower life expectancy than the general population.[2] Perhaps this last alarming statistic is due to another statistic: Female physicians appear to have a 3 to 4 times higher risk of suicide than do white females over the age of 35 in the general population.[4]

Compared to the general population, physicians also seem to be more prone to suffer certain behavioral and emotional problems. For example, Cooper et al[5] surveyed 1,817 general practitioners in England and found that, compared to the norms for the general male population, physicians scored significantly higher on measures of free-floating anxiety. Firth-Cozens[6,7] conducted a longitudinal study of 302 medical students who were in their fourth undergraduate year (1983 to 1984) and found that, at follow-up, 33% scored above threshold on a scale that measured symptoms of stress. In a 1997 study that employed the General Health Questionnaire,[8] Wall et al[9] found that 38% of British physicians polled evidenced "minor psychological problems" as compared to only 18% of workers outside the health care profession. And Olsen et al[10] reported that in today's milieu, physicians are likely to experience anger toward coworkers and patients, moodiness, fatigue, and mental distress.

For the past two decades, studies of physician well-being have also suggested that many physicians do a poor job of managing stress. For example, between 30% and 50% of physicians report anxiety, sleeplessness, or depression in reaction to personal problems,[11] percentages that are significantly higher than in other professions.[12] Approximately one-third of physicians polled reported recent incidents in which they considered their symptoms of stress as having negatively affected their delivery of patient care.[13] In some studies,[14] drug addiction and alcoholism were found to be 30 to 100 times more common in physicians than in the general population.

This academic debate aside, it is clear that to be a physician today is to be stressed. It therefore behooves any physician to periodically complete a stress assessment.

COPING AND STRESS SYMPTOMS

When it comes to stress management, if you are like most of us, you are a creature of habit. Stress hits, and you cope in predictable, over-learned ways. Your coping style is probably habitual: You tend to think, feel, relate to others, and behave automatically. Your individual coping steps are like dominoes lined on edge in a continuous stack. Each action, thought, or feeling tips the next. At some point in the progression, your stress symptoms surface. These are cues that something is bothering you and that it's time to disrupt at least one of the next steps in your typical coping progression.

Pattern disruption is a key factor in EEM. But this may be more difficult to do than it first appears. A dangerous tendency

EXERCISE 2-1

What Are Your Stress Symptoms?

Instructions: Check those symptoms and behaviors you typically experience either before, during, or after a stressful situation.

Physical Stress Symptoms

___Fast heart beats   ___Shallow breathing   ___Tense
                                                          shoulders/back

___Muscle twitching   ___Heartburn   ___Bowel problems

___Insomnia   ___Fatigue   ___Tearing eyes

___High blood pressure   ___Perspiring   ___Feeling flushed

___Dry mouth   ___Headaches   ___Backaches

___Jaw pain   ___Skin problems   ___Hives

___Excessive appetite   ___Loss of appetite

___Other_____

Stress Emotions

___Sad   ___Lonely   ___Angry

___Anxious   ___Disgusted   ___Contemptuous

___Manic   ___Energized   ___Fearful

___Discouraged   ___Helpless   ___Shy

___Paralyzed   ___Scattered   ___Numb

___Other_____

Stress Thinking

___Worrying   ___Worst-case thinking   ___Personalizing blame

___All-or-nothing   ___Selectively perceive   ___Difficulty focusing
                              negatives

___Difficulty concentrating ___Obsessive rumination   ___Angry thoughts

___Thoughts of persecution ___Self-pitying thoughts   ___Blaming others

___Other_____

Continued on next page

E X E R C I S E   2-1   (c o n t i n u e d)

Stress Behaviors

___Rushing	___Overworking	___Driving aggressively
___Slowing down	___Smoking	___Overusing alcohol
___Using illegal drugs	___Overeating	___Undereating
___Sleeping excessively	___Losing sleep	___Exercising excessively
___Becoming sedentary	___Achieving excessive escapism	___procrastinating

___Other_____

Interpersonal Behaviors

___Argumentative	___Controlling	___Competitive
___Defensive	___Sarcastic	___Bored
___Uncooperative	___Passive-aggressive	___Overly sensitive
___Unaffectionate	___Needy	___Unassertive, passive
___Aggressive	___Brusque	___Hurried

___Other_____

© 1999 Wayne and Mary Sotile.

---

shown by many high-performing copers is to go numb when stressed. We discuss this process more in our next chapter. Here, we simply want to emphasize that, although going numb may allow you to endure lengthy periods of stress, this same "talent" can also blunt your awareness of what your mind, body, or emotions are telling you at any given moment about your states of tension, fatigue, worry, or fear. Getting to know your own domino progression, or stress syndrome, is a prerequisite to healthy pattern disruption. So, let's start with a test (see Exercise 2-1).

As you read through the stress symptom checklist, keep a few things in mind. Some people show stress with physical symptoms: headaches, indigestion, chest pains, and so on. Some know they are stressed by their emotional reactions. They become angry, or anxious, or sad, or irritable. Others show stress in how they act. They make mistakes, can't sleep, forget things, and intensify their pace. For many, a major cause of stress is their coping style, in and of itself. For example, smokers might reach for cigarettes when stressed. Compulsive eaters might numb their anxiety by gorging themselves with food. Others run from stress into drug or alcohol abuse. Still others manifest stress in their dealings with the people around them. In each case, the method of *coping* with stress serves as another *source* of stress.

Now use Exercise 2-2 to summarize key observations from this self-assessment. First, note where you take stress "hits." Which of your *body systems* are most reactive to stress and strain?

If you had difficulty completing Exercise 2-2, observe yourself for several weeks, noticing how your body, emotions, thoughts, behaviors, and interactions tell you when you are building up stress. Think of these symptoms as being dominoes in your coping progression with red flags attached to them. By paying attention to these, you can learn important lessons about what stresses you and what you need to do right now to preserve your stress stamina.

Commit yourself to a 3-week period of self-observation. Take a minute four times each day to note your physical, emotional, cognitive, behavioral, and interpersonal stress symptoms. You might do this as you start your day (during your commute, for example), at noon, at mid-afternoon, and again early in the evening.

WHAT STRESSES YOU?

Once you begin to notice *when* you are stressed and *how* stress shows up, you are ready to fine-tune your understanding of the *causes* of your stress. We often start our stress management seminars with Exercise 2-3.

Most of us are tempted to draw the faces of *other people* in the space provided. Others answer by pointing out their most obvious aggravations. Still others note their most complex sources of stress, demons that have haunted them throughout life, for example, deeply embedded insecurities, wounds from past violations that simply won't heal, or deeply held fears.

The most difficult causes of stress share a common characteristic: They are aspects of life that are not under our direct and immediate control. Focusing on these will *not* improve your ability

E X E R C I S E 2-2

Self-Assessment Observations

Summarize your *physical* stress symptom responses in the following spaces.

My Body's Signs of Stress

_____

_____

_____

How do you *feel* when you are stressed? Note which adjectives you checked in the "Stress Emotions" subsection and summarize your observations below.

How I Feel When I Am Stressed

_____

_____

_____

Next, take note of how you tend to *think* when you are stressed. Summarize your "Stress Thinking" responses below.

How I Tend to Think When I Am Stressed

_____

_____

_____

How do you *behave* when you are stressed? In the spaces below, summarize your responses from the "Stress Behaviors" subsection.

How I Act When I Am Stressed

_____

_____

_____

Finally, note how you *treat others* when you are stressed. Summarize your observations from the "Interpersonal Behaviors" subsection.

How I Treat Others When I Am Stressed

_____

_____

_____

E X E R C I S E   2-3

What Stresses Me?

Instructions: In the spaces below, jot down your three major sources of stress.

_____

_____

_____

---

to manage your emotions. Doing so makes you more stressed, not more soothed. Another key to EEM is learning to focus your energies on managing what *is under your control* and avoid the tendency to overfocus on stresses that you cannot control. Plus, we have to avoid attempted solutions to our stresses that simply serve to perpetuate the very problems we are addressing. Here, you must beware of work addiction and compulsive working.

WORK ADDICTION

Long work hours and being a physician are synonymous. As we stated earlier, compared to other professionals, 3 times as many physicians spend 60 hours or more each week working.[15] Twenty-one percent work 80 hours per week and 16% work even longer hours.[16] However, work-addiction expert Bryan Robinson reminds us that working hard and being work addicted are not the same thing:

> "The major difference between abusive (or addictive) work and healthy (or constructive) work is the degree to which excessive work interferes with physical health, personal happiness or intimate and social relationships."[17 (p. 33)]

In *Beat Stress Together: How to Have a Passionate Marriage, a Healthy Family, and a Productive Life,*[18] we challenged what we termed the "myth of the balanced life" by asserting that, in truth, happy people who have successful families often work hard in jobs or careers they love. They enjoy their work and they're productive and effective in what they do. But they do not work to the point of *excluding* social and leisure activities, hobbies, and personal and family time.

Work abusers, on the other hand, do not control their compulsive work habits and feel unable to live up to both work responsibilities and family obligations. They lose perspective of any reasonable balance between work and other areas of their lives. They drive themselves beyond human endurance and put themselves under abnormal amounts of pressure by overdoing, overcommitting, and overcompensating.

Work addicts work for the sake of working and to gain the superficial, fleeting feelings of esteem and accomplishment that may come with work. Work addicts also avoid facing painful feelings by escaping into work and busyness; they overwork in an effort to fill a void that they can never fully satisfy. Because they are perfectionists, nothing is ever good enough for a work addict. So they keep trying to do more and better, believing that another accomplishment will make them complete. Because they chronically feel incomplete and unfinished, work addicts become dependent on overworking to gain a momentary positive sense of self-esteem. Finally, keeping the secret of work dependency is often part of the disease.

Robinson[17] organizes the major signs of work addiction around 10 broad categories that best describe the work addiction syndrome:

- *Hurrying and Staying Busy.* Work addicts are haunted by a constant sense of time urgency and are always struggling against the limits of time.

- *Need to Control.* Work addicts have an obsessive need to control themselves and others. This prevents them from asking for help or delegating responsibilities to others. As a result, they become overworked, tired, and overstressed.

- *Perfectionism.* Work addicts are such sticklers that they micromanage others and fail to discriminate important details from unimportant details. They are just as likely to be bothered by the grade of paper towels in the physicians' lounge as by the impact of government agencies on the practice of medicine. They hold high standards and judge both themselves and others accordingly.

- *Difficulty with Relationships.* Needless to say, excessive work can interfere with intimate relationships, close friendships, and collegiality with medical peers. Because all of their energies go into working compulsively, work abusers often appear to be inept and helpless in relationships. Spouses and family members of work addicts complain of being neglected, yet the work addict depends on others to manage the nonwork details of their lives, thereby freeing them to continue their overfocus on working. Yet, work addicts forget, ignore, or minimize important family rituals and celebrations, such as anniversaries, birthdays, or holidays. If they do participate, they bargain for trade-offs such as: "I'll go out to dinner with you on your birthday if you'll keep the kids out of my hair this week so I can finish my paper." If strong-armed into participating in a family function, the work addict does so dutifully but begrudgingly.

■ *Work Binges.* Robinson claims that the golden rule of the work addicted is, "Do today what doesn't need doing until six months from now."[17] (p. 52) Work addicts don't pace their work; they binge for days on a project until it is finished. Often, these binges are due to self-imposed early deadlines, not mandatory time frames. The sense of completion that comes from a binge is satisfying but simply leaves the work addict with time to focus on other work items. In advanced stages, work addiction leads to concealing work binges from friends and family, sneaking work when they get a chance. Some "pretend" that if they work when no family member is awake, it doesn't count as an inconvenience to anyone. They find themselves staying up later and rising earlier than their family members, just to have a binge of guilt-free overworking.

■ *Difficulty Relaxing and Having Fun.* Clearly, work addicts have difficulty turning off the nagging voice in their heads when they try to relax and unwind. When they do try to go on vacation or take a night off from work, they feel restless. They are likely to take work on vacation. While their family is sightseeing or playing on the beach, the work addict is back in the hotel room, alleviating work-driven anxieties. They confuse aversion relief with pleasure: "I feel great. I got all of the stuff that was bothering me on my 'to-do' list done. My headache is gone." That's not the same as having fun.

■ *Brownouts.* Mental preoccupation with planning and work keep work addicts out of the here and now. Friends and relatives may complain that the work addict may ask the same questions or tell the same stories several times. Some experience brownout while driving. They find themselves miles beyond the turn they intended to take and have no memory of how

they got there! Episodes of forgetfulness result from constant
mental planning and thinking about future work events.

■ *Impatience and Irritability.* Work addicts hate to be kept waiting,
and the world simply does not move fast enough for them.
They are easily annoyed at delays, lines, or inconveniences.
Many work addicts purposely arrive late for appointments, in
order to ensure that they will not waste time waiting.

■ *Self-Inadequacy.* Despite their accomplishments, addicted workers continue to feel badly about themselves. Work accomplishments only give them a temporary high. But no achievement is
ever enough. They continue to push themselves harder and
harder but continue to feel badly about themselves.

■ *Self-Neglect.* It is impossible to overwork, as addicts do without
engaging in self-neglect. A whole host of physical and emotional
problems may then result. These problems are compounded
when work addicts engage in poor health habits and are prone to
fuel their work binges with fast foods, caffeine, and nicotine, then
resort to some form of sedation, like alcohol, in an effort to "relax."

Do these notions apply to physicians? Often, the answer is yes.
Physicians have been found to rarely feel able to take time off
from work, even for physical problems.[19] In a study of Swedish
physicians,[3] 25% of physicians reported problems winding down
following a regular work day, a figure that was significantly
higher than for other professions. Further, one-third of the physicians polled by Arnetz reported that they regularly were too tired
to engage in social activities or to interact with their families, as
compared to only 10% for other employees.

Are You Work Addicted?

Robinson's work addiction risk test (WART)[20] (Exercise 2-4) can
help you measure your work compulsion.

Maybe You're Just Compulsive

In *Beat Stress Together*,[18] we elucidated the differences between
work addiction and compulsive working. We noted that Carter
and Carter have proposed that workaholics *prefer* work to interpersonal involvement. Compulsive workers, on the other hand,
are pushed to work by anxieties, excessive perfectionism, and

E X E R C I S E   2–4

The Work Addiction Risk Test

Instructions: Read each statement below and decide how much each one pertains to you. Using the rating scale, put the number that best fits you in the blank beside each statement.

1 ————— 2 ————— 3 ————— 4 ————— 5
never   sometimes   often   usually   always
true   true   true   true   true

Score:

___ 1. I prefer to do most things myself rather than ask for help.

___ 2. I get impatient when I have to wait for someone else or when something takes too long, such as long, slow-moving lines.

___ 3. I seem to be in a hurry and racing against the clock.

___ 4. I get irritated when I am interrupted while in the middle of something.

___ 5. I stay busy and keep many irons in the fire.

___ 6. I find myself doing two or three things at one time, such as eating lunch and writing a memo while talking on the phone.

___ 7. I overcommit myself by biting off more than I can chew.

___ 8. I feel guilty when I am not working on something.

___ 9. It is important that I see the concrete results of what I do.

___ 10. I am more interested in the final results of my work than in the process.

___ 11. Things just never seem to move fast enough or get done fast enough for me.

___ 12. I lose my temper when things don't go my way or work out to suit me.

___ 13. I ask the same question, without realizing it, after I've already been given the answer.

___ 14. I spend a lot of time mentally planning and thinking about future events, while tuning out the here and now.

___ 15. I find myself continuing to work after my coworkers have called it quits.

___ 16. I get angry when people don't meet my standards of perfection.

___ 17. I get upset when I cannot be in control of a situation.

Continued on next page

EXERCISE 2-4 (continued)

___ 18. I tend to put myself under pressure with self-imposed deadlines.

___ 19. It is hard for me to relax when I'm not working.

___ 20. I spend more time working than socializing with friends, on hobbies, or in leisure activities.

___ 21. I dive into projects to get a head start before all the phases have been finalized.

___ 22. I get upset with myself for making even the smallest mistake.

___ 23. I put more thought, time, and energy into my work than I do into my relationships with my partner, friends, and loved ones.

___ 24. I forget, ignore, or minimize important family celebrations such as birthdays, reunions, anniversaries, or holidays.

___ 25. I make important decisions before I have all the facts and have a chance to think them through thoroughly.

Compute your total score.

Total: _____

Scoring:
25–49 = You are not work addicted.
50–69 = You are mildly work addicted.
70–100 = You are highly work addicted.

©1998 Bryan Robinson. Used with permission.

---

their own discomfort with relaxing. According to the Carters, you might be a compulsive worker if you tend to work because you feel you have to, not because you love to. Following is a list of attitudes that tend to drive compulsive behaviors:

"It's better to stay at work and be caught up."

"I feel bored, guilty, and/or anxious if I'm not working."

"Anything worth doing is worth doing perfectly."

"There's not enough time for me to do all that I've committed to doing, so I'd better take advantage of every minute I can to chop away at this workload."

"You can't trust others to completely follow through. It's better to do it myself than to delegate responsibilities to others."

Regardless of what you call it, if your work style is one of the attempted solutions that is actually creating problems in your life, it's time to change. In many ways, overworking is a harder habit to kick than any other addiction because it is the only disease that draws applause from others. The task is to learn to separate abusive work habits from work effectiveness and become aware of the hidden motives for work dependency. Learn to not let work control you or your life.

SUBSTANCE ABUSE

No discussion of attempted solutions to stress problems would be complete without mention of substance abuse. Goldman et al[1] asserted that, contrary to popular beliefs, it is not true that physicians have higher absolute incidences of substance abuse than do members of the general population. However, no one would argue that physicians, like many high-performing professionals, are at risk of substance abuse. This concern is justified by studies that have shown that young physicians, especially, are at risk of depression and that there is a high co-morbidity between depression and alcoholism.[22] Specifically, Reuben[23] documented that, during the first year in practice, 29% to 38% of physicians are depressed. (These rates drop to 22% during the second year of practice and 10% in the third year.)

Our clinical experiences suggest that high-performing people are at risk of developing substance abuse problems because their drivenness compels them to work unless they are incapacitated. They have difficulty giving themselves permission to regularly engage in healthy, pleasurable activities. Intoxication provides a quick form of pseudo-relaxation and pleasure for someone who has difficulty otherwise experiencing these healing states.

A number of well-validated alcoholism screening scales are used in primary medical care settings.[24,25] Assess your own substance abuse potential by answering the 10 questions in Exercise 2-5.[26]

According to Ornstein and Sobel,[26] if you answered yes to any of these questions, drinking alcohol may be an unhealthy form of escape for you. If you answered yes to more than three questions, an alcohol problem is very likely. Seek professional help.

E X E R C I S E   2-5

Are You at Risk for Substance Abuse?

1. Do you have the following symptoms after drinking: stomach pain, nausea, heartburn, fatigue, weakness, frequent headaches, insomnia, or depression?

2. Do you need to drink in the morning to start the day?

3. Do you ever do things while drinking that you regret afterward?

4. Do you black out or forget what happened during a drinking episode?

5. Do you have trouble stopping drinking when you want?

6. Do you have five or more drinks daily?

7. Are your friends or family concerned about your drinking?

8. Does your drinking interfere with your family relationships or work?

9. Do you drive under the influence?

10. Do you have a family history of alcoholism?

CONCLUSIONS

The noted Stanford University physician John Farquhar[27] observed that ill health comes from small changes, each of which seems inconsequential in the moment. Positive health, too, results from small changes that add up to big differences. In this chapter, we have outlined a number of "small" choices that can help to create nurturing territory. But we recognize that many of us are driven by personality dynamics that compel us to behave in ways that defy good self-care. In our next chapter, we offer various perspectives on personality.

REFERENCES—CHAPTER 2

1. Goldman LS, Myers M, Dickstein LJ. Evolution of the physician health field. In: Goldman LS, Myers M, Dickstein LJ, eds. *The Handbook of Physician Health.* Chicago, Ill: American Medical Association; 2000:1–8.

2. Heim E. Job stressors and coping in health professions. *Psychother Psychosom.* 1991;55:90–99.

3. Arnetz BB. White collar stress: What studies of physicians can teach us. *Psychother Psychosom.* 1991;55:197–200.

4. Silverman MM. Physicians and suicide. In: Goldman LS, Myers M, Dickstein LJ, eds. *The Handbook of Physician Health.* Chicago, Ill: American Medical Association; 2000:95–117.

5. Cooper CL, Rout U, Faragher B. Mental health, job satisfaction, and job stress among general practitioners. *BMJ.* 1989;298:366–370.

6. Firth-Cozens J. Predicting stress in general practitioners: 10 year follow-up postal survey. *BMJ.* 1997;315:34–35.

7. Firth-Cozens J. Individual and organisational predictors of depression in general practitioners. *Br J Gen Prac.* 1998;1647–1651.

8. Goldberg D. *Manual of the General Health Questionnaire.* Windsor, UK: NFER; 1978.

9. Wall TD, Bolden RI, Borrill CS, Carter AJ, Golya DA, Hardy GE, Haynes CE, Rick JE, Shapiro DA, West MA. Minor psychiatric disorder in NHS trust staff: Occupational and gender differences. *Br J Psychiatry.* 1997;171:519–523.

10. Olsen RD, Sande JR, Olsen GP. Maternal parenting stress in physicians' families. *Clin Pediatr.* 1991;30:586–590.

11. Hendrie HC, Clair DK, Brittain HM, Fadul PE. A study of anxiety/depressive symptoms of medical students, house staff, and their spouses/partners. *J Nerv Ment Dis.* 1990;178:204–207.

12. Krakowski AJ. Stress and the practice of medicine: The myth and the reality. *J Psychosom Res.* 1982;26:91–98.

13. Firth-Cozens J, Greenhalgh J. Doctors' perceptions of the links between stress and lowered clinical care. *Soc Sci Med.* 44:1017–1022.

14. Domenighetti G, Tomamichel M, Gutzwiller F, Berthoud S, Casablanca A. Psychoactive drug use among medical doctors is higher than in the general population. *Soc Sci Med.* 1991;33:269–274.

15. Gross EB. Gender differences in physicians stress. *JAMWA.* 1992;47:107–114.

16. Fabri PJ, McDaniel MD, Gaskill HV, Garison RN, Hanks JB, Maier RV, Telford GL. Great expectations: Stress and the medical family. *J Surg Res.* 1989;47:379–382.

17. Robinson BE. *Work Addiction: Hidden Legacies of Adult Children.* Deerfield Beach, Fla: Health Communications, Inc; 1989.

18. Sotile WM, Sotile MO. *Beat Stress Together: The BEST Way to a Passionate Marriage, a Healthy Family, and a Productive Life.* New York, NY: Wiley & Sons; 1999.

19. McKevitt C, Morgan M, Dundas R, Holland WW. Sickness, absence and "working through" illness: A comparison of two professional groups. *J Public Health Med.* 1997;19:295–300.

20. Robinson B. *Chained to the Desk: A Guidebook for Workaholics, Their Partners and Children and the Clinicians Who Treat Them.* New York, NY: University Press; 1998.

21. Carter JM, Carter JD. *He Works/She Works™: Successful Strategies for Working Couples.* New York, NY: AMACOM; 1995.

22. British Medical Association, Working Group. *The Misuse of Alcohol and Other Drugs by Doctors.* London: British Medical Association; 1998.

23. Reuben DB. Depressive symptoms in medical house officers: Effects of level of training and work rotation. *Arch Intern Med.* 1985;145:286–288.

24. Ewing JA. Detecting alcoholism: The CAGE questionnaire. *JAMA.* 1984;252:1905–1907.

25. Powers JS, Spickard A. Michigan alcoholism screening test to diagnose early alcoholism in a general practice. *South Med J.* 1984;77:852–856.

26. Ornstein R, Sobel D. *Healthy Pleasures.* Reading, Mass: Addison-Wesley Publishing Co; 1989.

27. Faquhar J. *The American Way of Life Need Not Be Hazardous to Your Health.* New York, NY: Addison-Wesley Publishing Co; 1987.

The Psychology of Physicians

"Massive change in social roles has created new problems and has required new ways of coping with old problems."

C. M. Aldwin
*Stress, Coping, and Development:
An Integrative Perspective*[1] (p. 75)

If you are like most physicians, you probably live in a bitter-sweet, two-level paradox. The groundwork for the paradox started with your medical training, when you were taught to scan for the existence of pathology. This skill no doubt helps you to deliver competent medical care. But the habit of scanning for problems can interfere with your ability to accept yourself and others, flaws and all. That's the first level of the paradox.

Second, along the way of your medical training, you probably became proficient at self-denial—ignoring your feelings, your appetites, and your own needs—in order to get your job done and provide whatever is asked of you. Perhaps you entered medical school already prone to please others, even at your own expense. If not, you soon learned that doing so was a survival skill that allowed you to meet the extraordinary demands of medical training.

But this penchant for self-denial in order to care for others can be dangerous to your personal well-being. For example, researchers have cautioned that when medical training teaches you to repress awareness of your own needs and feelings and to rely too much on your ability to delay gratification as you work to gain approval from others, the result can be a life of struggling. What may follow is a lifestyle characterized by excessive busyness; compulsive pursuit of perfection; insistence that others submit to your way of doing things; emotional detachment; loss of playfulness; poor interpersonal relationships; and the "neurotic triad" of doubt, guilt, and exaggerated sense of responsibility.[2] The paradox: The very coping skills learned in your efforts to become a good caretaker serve to stress not only yourself but those around you.

IT'S NOT A SOLO DANCE

In Chapter 13, we show how empirical research has underscored the importance of physicians utilizing positive coping behaviors in the medical workplace and offer further guidelines for shaping the medical workplace into a positive interpersonal culture. In this chapter, we emphasize the flip side of this coin: How emotional *mismanagement* can become a physician's worst enemy. As depicted in Figure 3-1, mismanaged emotional reactions and counter reactions can result in self-perpetuating, circular dances between physicians and others who compromise outcomes, any way you care to measure them.[3]

Often, the deadly dance starts when the stressed physician reacts with mismanagement of his or her emotions. Next, the targets of the inappropriate physician behaviors respond to their own distress with passive and/or passive–aggressive behaviors. These, in turn, perpetuate further conflict. Soon, both parties are contributing to a self-perpetuating cycle of misery.

FIGURE 3-1

The Circular Dance of Misery

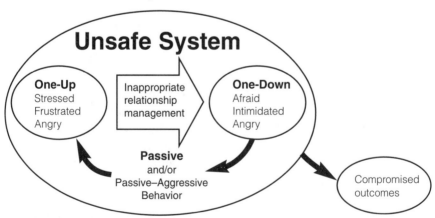

Source: Sotile WM, Sotile MO. Conflict Management: Part 1. How to shape positive relationships in medical practices and hospitals. The Physician Executive 1999;25(4):57-61. Used with permission.

This dance can take many forms. An intimidated nurse may cease asking for clarification of medical orders (a passive response), preferring to use her own medical judgment rather than risking another critical comment by an irritated physician. Passive reactions might also take a form that complicates medical staffing needs. We have observed health care professionals (including physicians) exercising passive control by missing work on days when the schedule dictates that they work closely with people who intimidate them or who otherwise make them uncomfortable.

Passive–aggressive reactions also come in various forms. Nurses may repeatedly "forget" a disruptive physician's desired protocols or medical orders, or a nurse may repeatedly find reasons to awaken certain physicians throughout a night of call duty. Still others may withhold information that would otherwise ease an offending physician's work.

Of course, nurses are not the only ones who can react to relationship tensions with passive–aggressive ploys; physicians sometimes deal with each other in this same manner. Examples include verbally or nonverbally criticizing another physician in front of patients, staff, colleagues, or referral sources; choosing to not respond or delay responding to calls from offending colleagues; refusing to participate in group meetings or practice management sessions; or misusing office or hospital equipment or practice resources, such as travel or continuing education allowances.[3]

Regardless of who "started it," all parties caught in such a swirl are stressed. Furthermore, we emphasize that no one can correct a strained relationship solo. But, just as we advise distressed individuals who seek our counsel for marital problems that their mates refuse to address, we encourage you to consider this fact: Even if only one partner in a dysfunctional "dance" changes his or her steps, the entire dance is altered. Doing so requires that you resist your temptation to respond to relationship tensions by dancing the steps that got you there, harder and faster. Rather, we recommend that you let relationship tensions serve as a wake-up call to look at your own contributions to the problems, rather than focusing on what the other person is doing or not doing. Start by examining your own personality and how you are driven to cope.

WHY DO YOU COPE AS YOU DO?

What drives me? Why am I compelled to cope in the ways I do? What can I do to make better coping choices? Questions like these haunt most thoughtful people. Of course, no ready-made answers can fully explain these phenomena. The existing theories about how personality develops and drives behavior differ drastically from each other. Further, no single theory is sacrosanct; many contradictory theories hold pearls of wisdom that are worth noting. In this chapter, we present key concepts from four schools of thought that we have found to be quite useful in our work with physicians interested in becoming more effective emotional managers. The four theories to be discussed are: the psychodynamic perspective; the integrative, coping perspective; the transactional analysis perspective; and an interpersonal perspective on Type A behavior patterns.

Psychodynamic Perspective

Psychodynamic theory proposes that the emotions of anxiety, shame, guilt, sadness, anger, and sexual arousal play particularly important roles in driving our behavior.[4] Such feelings are said to create conflicts that serve either consciously or through our unconscious to fuel certain modes of adapting. Classic psychodynamic theorists such as Horney[5,6] proposed that psychic conflicts lead to needs that are expressed in ways that serve to defend against what would happen if underlying feelings were openly expressed (summarized by Kilburg[4]). Examples of how this perspective might explain certain aspects of your coping style follow. As you read through these examples, note how a basic human fear can lead to a personality adaptation that fuels a style of living that suggests an underlying need.

- Fears of self-assertion, conflict, or hostility in self or others may lead to an exaggerated *need for affection and approval*, which may compel you to indiscriminately conform to the wishes of others.
- Fears of abandonment and being alone may fuel *the need for a partner to adore and be admired by*, thereby driving you to prove yourself to be loveable by taking on the role of self-denying rescuer.

- Fears of self-expression and making demands may lead to *the need to restrict your life within narrow borders.* This may result in quashed ambition, remaining in second place (eg, "the eternal resident" mentality), and adoption of excessive modesty as the supreme value. For such individuals, difficulty saying no and setting limits when responding to the demands of others can lead to a psychic exhaustion that borders on depression.

- Fear of mistakes, errors, bad judgment, loss of control or helplessness, and of any limits to one's own ability to control others may lead to *an exaggerated need for power.* These people try to dominate all things and all relationships. Their combativeness, basic disrespect for other's feelings and dignity, and contempt for weakness of any kind (in self and others) make them stern taskmasters who tend to drive others away. Their open adoration of strength and their belief in the omnipotence of intelligence and reason fuel a hyperresponsiveness to any frustration.

- Fears of being exploited and possessed may fuel *a need to exploit others.* These individuals pride themselves on their ability to manipulate, exploit, or possess others. They treat other people like objects to be used for their own gains.

- Fear of public humiliation or shame can lead to *an excessive need for social recognition or prestige.* Here, self-esteem is based disproportionately on social acceptance. In its exaggerated form, this dynamic may compel a person to act narcissistically entitled; as though life is about being admired for one's fantasy image of oneself.

- Fears of failure and low self-esteem may fuel *an excessive need for personal achievement.* Here, self-worth is dependent on being recognized as "the best." Life becomes a constant striving to compete and defeat others. The relentless, anxiety-based drive for success that characterizes this pattern may result in workaholism.

- Some people mask their fears of attachment, love, or needing others by showing *a distorted need for self-sufficiency and independence.* Staying detached from others becomes a major source of security. Belonging to a team or group, on the other hand, stirs primitive insecurities that may lead to behaviors that sabotage one's team membership.

■ Fears of public humiliation or shame may fuel *a need for perfection*. Errors, mistakes, flaws, or criticism become anathema for such people, and their lack of self-acceptance makes them critical taskmasters in their dealings with others.

Splitting

Another useful psychodynamic explanation of how unrequited needs fuel personality development hinges on the concept of splitting. Based on the peculiarities of the formative influences in our lives, we are each taught to feel uncomfortable with certain ways of behaving, thinking, or feeling that otherwise would become a natural, healthy part of our behavioral and emotional repertoire. As a result, each of us develops an internal psychological "splitting" that lurks at the core of our sense of self. One part of the split contains the characteristics that please those around us, based on *their* needs, not ours. We are taught that these are admirable aspects of self. We quickly learn that expressing these "good self" traits inspires a positive outcome. These behaviors, thoughts, or feelings will allow us to either gain pleasure and acceptance or avoid pain and rejection. On the other hand, any thoughts, feelings, needs, or wants that meet with disapproval, discomfort, or shaming from significant others get repressed and stored in the unexpressed or "bad" aspect of self.

Because we are motivated to avoid pain and gain pleasure, we tend to fill our lives with choices that further our internal splits. We over-express our "good" traits and under-express our "bad" ones. In the process of doing so, we increase our familiarity and comfort with the components of our expressed self, but we are left with festering, lingering doubts and discomfort about the thoughts, feelings, and needs that are in our unexpressed self. In this way, a split develops between the expressed and unexpressed selves.

If the split is extreme, personality disorders develop. Such people tend to be filled with rage that is stored in the unexpressed self; often, their anger masks hurts that came from abuse or neglect at the hands of narcissistic or uncaring caretakers or other significant authority figures.

At minimum, these "split-off" aspects of self tend to lead to chronic distress that stirs defensive reactions and fuels certain flavors of drivenness. Internal psychological splitting and conflicts create psychic pain that must be defended against.

Defenses

Kilburg[4] succinctly summarized the mechanisms of psychological defense that leaders in the field[7-9] have proposed. These include the following:

- *Primitive mechanisms:* Defenses often seen in psychosis, dreams, and normal childhood. Examples include denial, splitting, distortion, and delusional projection.
- *Immature mechanisms:* Seen in severe depression, personality disorders, and adolescence. Examples include fantasy, projection, passive–aggressive behavior, hypochondriasis, dissociation, derealization, and acting out (criminality, sadism, perversion).
- *Neurotic mechanisms:* Defenses common in everyone, including intellectualization, repression, reaction formation, displacement, dissociation, and detachment.
- *Mature mechanisms:* Commonly seen in healthy adults, these defenses include sublimation, altruism, suppression, anticipation, humor, curiosity, creativity, constructive work and play, reality testing, problem-solving, wisdom, love, communication skills, and accurate empathy.

The major purpose for psychological defenses is to avoid pain and suffering and to create at least the illusion of control over your psychological realm. Often, defensiveness leads to complex patterns of interpersonal behaviors, like relationship game-playing and rituals that are fueled by the cognitive distortions that stem from the notion that it would be unsafe to openly disclose one's true self when dealing with others. The drama that fuels defensive behavior is the fear that open expression of one's vulnerabilities and needs will result in pain, punishment, or humiliation, rather than in nurturance.

The Psychodynamics of Physicians

The psychodynamic perspective on physician behavior has pivoted around the findings from a famous longitudinal study of physicians conducted by George Vaillant and colleagues.[10] These researchers found that the physicians who became casualties of the rigors of medical training and practice were those who *entered* the profession suffering from fundamental insecurities, low self-esteem, emotional dependency, social anxiety, and a tendency toward depression. This finding was replicated in subsequent studies that suggested that, of those physicians who committed suicide, approximately 40% brought symptoms of emotional and psychological problems with them into medical training, while 60% got symptomatic in reaction to the stresses and strains of medical education and practice.[11,12]

Psychodynamically oriented theorists have further proposed that vulnerable physicians suffered childhoods lacking in adequate emotional nurturance from parental figures. The result? They learned to repress awareness of their own needs and feelings[2,13] and to delay gratification of their own needs and steadfastly work to gain approval from others.

Others observed that some physicians become so preoccupied with their own frustrations that they appear to be "pathologically narcissistic."[14] Still others have proposed that many physicians respond to their unfulfilled desire for an intimate and loving parental relationship by adopting an endless quest to gain respect from colleagues and community. As they go about trying to be all things to all people, daily fixes of adoration and appreciation from patients create the opportunity to give to others what was never received as a child.[2,10]

These psychological factors, coupled with the relentless demands of medical education and practice, may result in solidification of what researchers Gabbard and Menninger termed *the hallmark psychological characteristics of physicians:* compulsiveness, perfectionism, insistence that others submit to their way of doing things, emotional detachment, doubt, guilt, an exaggerated sense of responsibility, and an excessive devotion to work and productivity to the exclusion of pleasure and value of interpersonal relationships.[2,15] Johnson[14] proposed that these same psychodynamics may contribute to poor self-care and to a vulnerability to substance abuse and depression in physician populations.

Even those who are skeptical about psychodynamic explanations of physician behavior tend to agree that many physicians suffer a personal sense of emotional impoverishment that stems from the effects of perfectionism and the self-sacrificing that is part of a life of care-taking.[16,17] This combination of psychological traits is likely to fuel chronic self-doubt and guilt as to whether or not enough has been done to satisfy and please others. Unfortunately, research has shown that physicians who are highly self-critical show significantly increased levels of stress and depression.[18] The aforementioned study by McCranie and Brandsma[19] demonstrated how the combination of low self-esteem, feelings of inadequacy, dysphoria and obsession, worry, passivity, social anxiety, and withdrawal predispose physicians to increased burnout.

AN INTEGRATIVE, COPING PERSPECTIVE

In our opinion, a true understanding of an individual's psychology requires a broadening of the psychodynamic perspective. Contemporary theorists have noted that much of personality development comes from interactions with significant others beyond the mother–father–child triad[1] and that psychological development progresses throughout adult life.[20] In *Stress, Coping, and Development,* University of California, Davis, researcher Carolyn Aldwin, PhD, offered a pithy description of the cornerstone concept in the integrative coping perspective:

> "Rather than a person's 'adaptational style' being 'set in stone' due to genetics or fixation at early stages of personality development, coping strategies are thought to be plastic, to develop in the course of dealing with the ever-changing stress in the environment."[1 (p. 216)]

Aldwin goes on to brilliantly summarize two decades of research by way of arguing that coping is a fluid process, influenced by personality characteristics, situational demands, and the social and physical characteristics of the setting. The integrative coping perspective holds that the crucial factor in understanding one's coping style is the "goodness of fit" between the demands of a situation, the capacities of an individual, and the quality of the interpersonal context in which the coping takes place.[21] Your early life experiences are seen to be but one of several factors that shape personality. The pulls of your current environment and the people in it, the status of your contemporary relationships, and the choices you make in responding to your current developmental challenges will have much to do with your stress resilience. This perspective also proposes that, regardless of the sources of your conflicts, the final common pathway between what happens *to* us and how we feel is how we cope.

The coping challenge faced by physicians is to learn flexibility. The difficulty of doing so is captured in the study of emotion-focused and problem-focused coping styles. As summarized by Aldwin,[1] *problem-focused coping* is an attempt to control or manage a stressful situation. This style of coping is particularly effective when facing stressors that can, indeed, be changed. Longitudinal studies[22] have shown that taking charge with problem-focused coping decreases psychological symptoms of stress and increases a feeling of mastery when facing controllable situations.

This style of coping certainly has its advantages. Problem-focused copers tend to be optimistic[23] and less neurotic[24] than individuals who show predominant use of other coping styles. And problem-focused coping leads to an increased sense of control when facing a *controllable* stressor. For example, many work problems must be resolved by addressing them directly, taking charge of the problem, and eliminating or solving it. The same is true when dealing with controllable risk factors that perpetuate many disease states, things like smoking cigarettes, unhealthy eating, or high-risk sexual practices.

But active, problem-focused coping has negative consequences when it is *misapplied.* For example, if used when facing an *uncontrollable* stressor, active coping actually *increases* emotional distress and may also increase blood pressure and general cardiovascular response.[25] And attempting to control another person may prove to be fruitless and frustrating for you as well as damaging to your relationship.

When the stressor is uncontrollable, a different kind of coping is called for—a coping style that baffles many physicians. It's called emotion-focused coping. *Emotion-focused coping* relies on cognitive efforts (like rationalization or denial) to *reinterpret* the situation in some way, rather than sheer will of force to *change* the situation. This sort of coping is sometimes termed *avoidant coping.* In contrast to the approach strategies that characterize problem-focused coping, emotion-focused coping has been shown to lower symptoms of stress when facing situations like the death of a loved one, a disappointing setback, or the need for surgery—situations that are uncontrollable.[26, 27] Here, coping strategies, like denial, which might typically be considered antithetical to psychological health, help, at least in the short term.[1] Emotion-focused coping can also help to ease the frustration that comes when another person fails to conform to your expectations.

Given the foregoing facts, consider the plight of a physician faced with this question: Should I fight (problem-focused coping) the managed care movement that is changing the practice of medicine or should I find a way to accept this and maximize my comfort in the process (emotion-focused coping)?

We, of course, cannot answer this question for you. But we do believe that here, as in general, the point is to develop coping flexibility. When evaluating "good" and "bad" coping, consider what the situation demands and the relative costs and benefits of different coping strategies. Each mode of coping has its advantages. Avoidant strategies have been shown to be more effective in reducing emotional distress in the short term; approach strategies are more effective over the long run.[28] Choose how you cope respecting your own quality of life and individual goals. Otherwise, you will be left feeling helpless and hopeless rather than developing a sense of coping self-efficacy.

One final thought: The managed care dilemma calls to mind the final sage words of Aldwin[1] who reminds us that:

"Social activists (problem-focused copers) may do the society as a whole a great deal of good. But, in the short-run, they may suffer increased psychological and physical distress for themselves (and perhaps for their families as well)."[(p. 168)]

Coping Patterns And Pitfalls

In *The Medical Marriage,* we proposed a simple conceptualization of coping patterns and pitfalls.[29] This model is based on transactional analysis theory,[30] which asserts, in part, that six coping themes tend to drive our ways of thinking, behaving, and feeling. Some combination of the following "drivers" typically shapes both our stress reactions and our relationship dynamics: Being Strong, Being Perfect, Trying Hard, Pleasing Others, Hurrying, and Being Careful.

Being Strong
If you were taught that your role in life is to be strong and stoic, never complaining about your pains and fears, you probably are driven by a Being Strong personality theme. You are likely to have trouble asking for support and help during hard times. You may even have trouble noticing when you need help because you have split off awareness of feelings such as vulnerability and fear. Instead, you selectively attend to more "powerful" feelings, such as anger. The result can be loneliness as you go through life numbing your emotional awareness and quietly facing your stressors.

Being Perfect

If you are driven by a Being Perfect coping theme, you are probably quite accustomed to feeling anxious, irritable, and guilty.
Because perfection is impossible to attain or sustain, you likely
spend much of your time fussing: at others for their shortcomings
and at yourself for your own blemishes.

Trying Hard

Some of us learn to equate self-worth with fatigue. We have been
taught that our special value lies in our ability to struggle longer
and harder with the tasks and obligations that fill our lives than
others. If you are driven by a Trying Hard coping style, you may
have difficulty determining when you have worked hard enough
to deserve a rest and you probably feel anxious when you try to
relax or play. You deal with stress by narrowly focusing on the
tasks at hand—relentlessly pursuing your goals and only resting
once your ignored fatigue builds into exhaustion.

Pleasing Others

If you have difficulty being appropriately self-focused and self-
nurturing without feeling guilty, you are probably driven by a
Pleasing Others coping style. Such folks have difficulty saying no
to requests from others and equal difficulty figuring out their
own needs and wants. Even when you are aware of what you
need or want, you probably have difficulty asking directly. This
self-sacrificing way of living is exhausting. Brief periods of withdrawal and depression become indirect ways of gaining relief
from the constant push to be a caretaker. Unfortunately, rather
than rejuvenating, these periods of withdrawal tend to fuel guilt
and anxiety, which may catapult you into another Pleasing
Others flurry.

Hurrying

Some of us were taught to rush through life. If you are driven by
a Hurrying coping style, you probably live with an internal sense
of urgency. When forced to slow down (by health problems, the
"slowness" of others, or your own limitations), you are likely to
suffer anxiety, frustration, and irritability.

TABLE   3-1

Signs of Personality-Based Stress

If you cope rigidly by:	Then your stress symptom is likely to be:
Being strong	Loneliness and numbness
Trying hard	Fatigue and joylessness
Pleasing others	Guilt, anxiety, and withdrawal
Being perfect	Guilt, irritability, and obsessing
Being careful	Fear and difficulty making decisions
Hurrying	Anxiety and urgency

Being Careful

If you often feel free-floating anxiety—scared and anxious but unaware of what is bothering you—you probably learned to cope by Being Careful. You may obsessively worry about worst-case scenarios. On an emotional level, these imagined outcomes begin to feel real. Being Careful causes high levels of anxiety, especially when you are faced with the need to make decisions. You worry about the potential consequences of decisions, your own or those made by loved ones. In short, you often plague yourself (and your loved ones) with your paralyzing fear of change.

Patterns and Pitfalls Cycles

Each of these ways of coping can be helpful; each works some-times in some situations. But, coping problems develop when we rigidly lock into overusing our most familiar driver. As shown in Table 3-1, the signs that your coping efforts are not fully working to soothe you emotionally can come in various forms, depending upon your personality scripting.

Looking over Table 3-1, you can see that symptoms of stress vary depending upon your coping style. Different people know they are stressed when they feel numb, or fatigued, or with-drawn, or irritated, or afraid. This is an important point, especial-ly for high-powered people who tend to discount the notion that stress affects them. We often make the mistake of assuming that if we are not acting like "nervous wrecks," we must not be stressed. As we discuss later, high-powered people tend to be driven by

T A B L E   3-2

Coping Patterns and Underlying Hopes

Driver	Underlying Hope
Being Strong	To be nurtured
Being Perfect	To feel good enough
Trying Hard	To feel deserving of rest and enjoyment
Pleasing Others	To feel understood and appreciated
Hurrying	To feel finished
Being Careful	To feel safe

personality programming that short-circuits anxiety. If you are like most physicians we have known, your stress symptoms are more likely to be feelings of loneliness, numbness, guilt, fatigue, irritability, or urgency—anything but anxiety.

Table 3-2 shows how the behaviors that come with each of the personality drivers usually mask underlying hopes and needs. For example, the hope underlying being strong is the wish to be nurtured. Unfortunately, clinical experience suggests that physicians and other high-performing people tend to ignore their own and each other's underlying needs. Our driver behaviors make this easy to do. Let us elaborate.

When we act strong, for example, we convey the message that we do not need anything from anyone. Our underlying need—to be nurtured—may therefore go unsoothed. The more unsoothed we feel, the more we tend to drive ourselves with the original driver pattern.

Eventually, we end up stuck in a coping pitfall characterized by the stress symptoms outlined in Table 3-1. As shown in Table 3-1, high-powered people driven by a need to be strong end up feeling lonely and numb, the antithesis of the nurturance needed.

Often, a vicious cycle ensues; a cycle that can last a lifetime and that can thwart both individual well-being and growth in any relationship. As we drive ourselves harder and harder, we continue to misrepresent our underlying needs and therefore continue to experience the frustration of not getting these underlying needs met. Soon, we lose sight of the part we are playing in perpetuating our own discomfort and we misinterpret our driver-caused pain as an indication that something is wrong with the people around us. We then cycle back and forth between acting out our driver patterns, accumulating pain, displacing and projecting blame onto others, growing ever-more frustrated, and driving harder and harder.

Eventually, you may begin to believe that other people are the *cause* of your distress. What an unnecessary tragedy! This pattern is fueled by a simple factor that can ruin relationships: lack of a clear understanding of your own and other's underlying needs.

Use the information in Tables 3-1 and 3-2 as guides and reminders. When you notice yourself feeling or acting in ways that are suggested in the stress symptoms column of Table 3-1, ask for input that might soothe your corresponding underlying hope described in Table 3-2. For example, if you find yourself feeling exhausted and joyless, it may be that you are hurting yourself by staying stuck in a Trying Hard driver. You may be having difficulty giving yourself permission to take your fair share of rest and enjoyment. Asking for supportive input and "permission" from a trusted loved one as a reminder to you that you do, indeed, deserve your fair share of rest and enjoyment will make it easier to do what you need to do to recuperate your energies.

Similarly, if you notice a loved one acting in ways suggested in the stress symptoms column of Table 3-1, you can use this information to help structure a more nurturing reaction. First, assume that your loved one is suffering frustration of the corresponding underlying hope (see Table 3-2). Next, offer a nurturing "gift" that might soothe that underlying hope. For example, if your partner is obsessing and preoccupied with feelings of guilt and anxiety, you might offer encouragement that he or she is making good enough progress in dealing with the problem at hand, even though no perfect outcome has yet occurred. Or, you might offer words of reassurance and calming if your partner is acting fearful and worrying without any specific focus to his or her concerns.

If you learn to directly identify and soothe your own and others' underlying hopes and needs, you will accomplish two important tasks. First, you will disrupt the aforementioned tendency to "go numb" and gradually burn out. Second, if you soothe another's underlying needs—rather than lock into a "posturing" struggle in response to the other's stress symptom (a topic discussed in Chapter 8)—you will serve as a source of resilience for that person. The result will be a more flexible, safe, collaborative, even loving (if appropriate) relationship.

Type A Pattern Behavior

Our clinical experiences suggest that stress leads many physicians to develop a high-powered coping style that may serve them well in the moment but that magnifies preexisting coping tendencies to problem proportions. It's called Type A behavior pattern (TYABP).

What Is TYABP? Cardiologists Meyer Friedman and Ray Rosenman originated the concept of TYABP from their observations that their hard-driving heart patients often seemed stuck in a lifestyle of struggling: They aggressively struggled to achieve more and more in less and less time, and they justified their struggling with the world view that the environment is a hostile or limiting place filled with incompetent people.[31] Furthermore, they seemed convinced that other people were invested in opposing their progress, a perception that further justified their constant struggling.

We emphasize that TYABP does not refer to a set personality *trait;* it is a multifaceted construct. It is a *way of coping* that consists of many factors, at least some of which will emerge in *any* person who is placed in the wrong situation long enough.[32] Some people develop certain aspects of TYABP and others do not; some show TYABP in certain situations and not in others.

Table 3-3 is a list of psychological and behavioral characteristics that have been earmarked by contemporary researchers as typifying the Type A coping style.[33] We hope that you will use this information to empower yourself to take more nurturing control of yourself and of your relationships, not to blame or shame.

As you read through the list, check descriptions that apply to you or to a loved one, colleague, or associate. Also, note the situations that are most likely to stir your Type A reactions. And remember: These are general characteristics of TYABP; the list is not exhaustive. Note what needs to be added or subtracted from the list to accurately describe *your* coping style.

If you are stuck in a Type A style of coping—or in a relationship with someone with TYABP—you will relate to the words of Canadian psychologist Ethel Roskies. Perhaps more than

T A B L E   3-3

Summary of Type A Response Styles

The Type A individual is driven by:

Conscientiousness and an inflexible sense of responsibility

Perfectionism

High levels of cynicism and hostility

The need to prove self-worth by performing well

Cravings for recognition and power

Competition and challenges

Driving need to work long, hard hours

The desire to be seen as a leader

A vague mistrust of the motives or competency of others

Type A behaviors include:

Tense, energetic movements

Constant movement: Difficulty being still, fidgeting, tapping feet, drumming knuckles, or shaking leg or foot while attempting to sit still

Explosively emphasizing points with finger and hand motions during conversation

Frequent uses of profanity

Forceful expressions of opinions, often using such words as "stupid," "idiotic," and "ridiculous" in response to opinions differing from one's own

Flashing grimace-like smiles

A clipped speaking pattern, the result of constantly tensing jaw muscles

Irregular breathing pattern, often leading to expiratory sighs in the midst of conversations

Constant rushing and fighting against time, also known as hurry sickness

Overly aggressive and competitive reactions even when the situation does not warrant such

Doing several things at once

TABLE 3-3 (continued)

The Type A's style and focus of thinking:

Tends to think on several levels at once

Anticipates what is coming next and reacts in advance (eg, interrupts conversations with answers to unfinished questions or prepares for departure from car or airplane well before the vehicle stops)

Hypervigilant: Scans surroundings, noticing what might go wrong or what is irritating at the moment

Constantly checks the time, noting time crunch, punctuality (own or others'), and efficiency (or lack thereof)

Preoccupation with all of the above, resulting in poor observational abilities, especially of one's own behavior or of the impact of one's own behavior on others

Factors that affect interpersonal relationships for Type As:

Self-focused: Preoccupied with own stresses, anxieties, or tasks

Poor listener: Interrupts, breaks rapport with distracted behavior, gives advice rather than empathy

Easily bored by another's conversation

Easily angered and has difficulty not showing it (glaring, curt comments, or honking the horn at others while driving)

Makes critical, blaming, or shaming comments when someone makes a mistake

Defensive in reacting to feedback, especially regarding obvious hostility

Shows overt bravado and confidence regarding own opinions, abilities, and power

Often frustrated when working with others

Very controlling: Dictates, gives unsolicited advice

Visibly uncomfortable with physical intimacy or verbal expressions of tender feelings

Source: Sotile WM. *Heart Illness and Intimacy: How Caring Relationships Aid Recovery.* Baltimore, Md, Johns Hopkins University Press; 1992. Adapted with permission.

anything, Roskies[34] proposes, TYABP is an *inefficient use of powerful coping energy.* As she puts it:

> The Type A is more often at war than at peace, repeatedly mobilizing his or her resources to confront perceived threats and challenges. A game of tennis, a difference of opinion with a colleague at work, and a too-slow elevator all produce a stress reaction in the hypersensitive Type A. . . . Even a nonstressful environment [will] be perceived and reacted to as challenging by the hyper-reactive Type A. There are no safe environments for the person who engages in mortal combat even during a "friendly" game of tennis!

TYABP will magnify any of the personality-based driver patterns described earlier. For example:

- The stress-hardy individual whose Being Strong personality typically serves him or her well can go numb in an ever-escalating flurry of Type A reactivity.
- As TYABP gets more intense, the orderly are at risk of becoming compulsively driven toward Being Perfect behavior.
- The relentless drive to achieve what comes with TYABP can push Trying Hard tendencies into workaholism.
- The Type A-driven need for approval from others can lead the typically Pleasing Others person to live as though life is a quest to be all things to all people.
- The hurry sickness inherent in TYABP can propel a person already scripted to Hurrying into a lifestyle of free-floating anxiety and irritability.
- The typically cautious person can become quasi-paranoid as his or her Type A-driven anxieties amplify his Being Careful personality scripting.

Parker and Jones,[35] in a study of dual-physician Australian couples, made the point that a medical career attracts overt or latent Type A individuals and then promotes such characteristics in them. However, few well-controlled research studies regarding TYABP and physicians have been published. Naser et al[36] claimed that TYABP is more prevalent in surgeons, pediatricians, and OB/GYNs than in psychiatrists. Women physicians have been found to be much more likely to evidence Type A coping patterns than are either male physicians or women who are not physicians.[37,38]

F I G U R E   3-2

Paradigm for Developing Coping Problems

Repress your own needs
+
Delay gratification as a lifestyle
+
Work obsessively at gaining approval
+
Make excessive use of problem-focused coping
+
Develop an inflated persona
and/or
Try Hard, Please Others, and Be Perfect drivers
+
Live in high-demand/low-control stress paradigms

LEADS TO

Workaholism
+
Neurotic triad:
-Doubt
-Guilt
-Exaggerated sense of responsibility
+
TYABP

Which fuels

Interpersonal tensions at work
(interact circularly)
Interpersonal tensions at home

LEADS TO

High demand/low control/low support
(cycles back up to repressing own needs or to inflated persona and/or
Try Hard, Please Others)

HOW PHYSICIANS DEVELOP COPING PROBLEMS

None of the perspectives on coping explained thus far is universally applicable. However, we believe that each of these perspectives lends something of value in understanding how coping problems can develop for physicians. Figure 3-2, modified from Gabbard,[2] integrates key points from the foregoing discussions into a paradigm for developing coping problems. It presents a set of guidelines for what *not* to do.

CONCLUSIONS

We close this chapter with the reminder that, regardless of what drives you or what you face, your hope for health and happiness lies in the fact that you are not a passive responder. Your coping style consists of learned behaviors, and you can develop new coping habits. We hope that the various perspectives we offered about personality styles and patterns have stirred your thinking about the costs and benefits of your own coping habits.

If you are like most of us, you achieve greater levels of self-satisfaction and well-being when you periodically change aspects of yourself, your environment, and your relationships. The good news of our EEM model is that, when it comes to managing the net effects of your coping styles, *little changes make big differences.*

However, it is also true that sustaining high levels of well-being requires that you commit to periodically modifying the choices that are shaping your coping style, your lifestyle, and your interpersonal dynamics. Herein lies the hard work of stress-hardy living. This task is made easier if you become familiar with several paradigms that can help to organize your efforts to change and grow. We turn next to discussion of this important topic.

REFERENCES—CHAPTER 3

1. Aldwin CM. *Stress, Coping, and Development: An Integrative Perspective.* New York, NY: Guilford; 1994.
2. Gabbard GO. The role of compulsiveness in the normal physician. *JAMA.* 1985;254:2926–2929.
3. Sotile WM, Sotile MO. Conflict management: Part 1. How to shape positive relationships in medical practices and hospitals. *The Physician Executive.* 1999;25:57–61.
4. Kilburg RR. *Executive Coaching: Developing Managerial Wisdom in a World of Chaos.* Washington, DC: American Psychological Association; 2000.
5. Horney K. *The Neurotic Personality of Our Time.* New York, NY: W.W. Norton; 1937.
6. Horney K. *Self Analysis.* New York, NY: W.W. Norton; 1942.
7. Valliant GE. *Adaptation to Life.* Boston, Mass: Little, Brown; 1977.
8. Conte JR, Plutchik R, eds. *Ego Defenses: Theory and Measurement.* New York, NY: John Wiley & Sons; 1995.
9. Berne E. *Games People Play: The Basic Handbook of Transactional Analysis.* New York, NY: Ballantine; 1964.
10. Valliant GE, Sobowale NC, McArthur C. Some psychologic vulnerabilities of physicians. *N Engl J Med.* 1972;287:372–375.
11. Roy A. Suicide in doctors. *Psychiatr Clin North Am.* 1985;8:377–387.
12. Krakowski AJ. Stress and the practice of medicine: The myth and the reality. *J Psychosom Res.* 1982;26:91–98.
13. Menninger K. Psychological factors in the choice of medicine as a profession. *Bull Menninger Clin.* 1957;21:51–58, 99–106.
14. Johnson WDK. Predisposition to emotional distress and psychiatric illness amongst doctors: The role of unconscious and experiential factors. *Br J Med Psychol.* 1991;64:317–329.
15. Gabbard GO, Menninger RW. The psychology of postponement in the medical marriage. *JAMA.* 1989;261:2378–2381.
16. Gabbard GO, Menninger RW. *Medical Marriages.* Washington, DC: American Psychiatric Press, Inc; 1988.
17. Gautam M. Depression and anxiety. In: Goldman LS, Myers M, Dickstein LJ, eds. *The Handbook of Physician Health.* Chicago, Ill: American Medical Association; 2000:80–94.

18. Firth-Cozens J. Predicting stress in general practitioners: 10 year follow up postal survey. *BMJ.* 1997;315:34–35.

19. McCranie EW, Brandsma JM. Personality antecedents of burnout among middle-aged physicians. *Behav Med.* 1988;(Spring):30–36.

20. Levinson DJ. *The Seasons of a Man's Life.* New York, NY: Ballantine; 1978.

21. Coyne J, Smith DAF. Couples coping with a myocardial infarction: A contextual perspective on wives' distress. *J Pers Soc Psychol.* 1991; 61:404–412.

22. Pearlin LI, Lieberman MA, Menaghan EG, Mullan JT. The stress process. *J Health Soc Behav.* 1981;22:337–356.

23. Long BC, Sangster JI. Dispositional optimism/pessimism and coping strategies: Predictors of psychosocial adjustment of rheumatoid and osteoarthritis patients. *J Appl Soc Psychol.* 1993;23:1069–1091.

24. Bolger N. Coping as a personality process: A prospective study. *J Pers Soc Psychol.* 1990;59:525–537.

25. Dolan CA, Sherwood A, Light KC. Cognitive coping strategies and blood pressure responses to real-life stress in healthy young men. *Health Psychol.* 1992;11:233–242.

26. Mattlin J, Wethington E, Kessler RC. Situational determinants of coping and coping effectiveness. *J Health Soc Behav.* 1990;31:103–122.

27. Vitaliano PP, DeWolfe DJ, Maiuro RD, Russo J, Karon W. Appraisal changeability of a stressor as a modifier of the relationship between coping and depression: A test of the hypothesis of fit. *J Pers Soc Psychol.* 1990;59:582–592.

28. Mullen B, Suls J. The effectiveness of attention and rejection as coping styles: A meta-analysis of temporal differences. *J Psychosom Res.* 1982;26:43–49

29. Sotile WM, Sotile MO. *The Medical Marriage: Sustaining Positive Relationships for Physicians and Their Families.* Revised Edition. Chicago, Ill: American Medical Association Press; 2000.

30. Stewart I, Joines V. *TA Today: A New Introduction to Transactional Analysis.* Nottingham, England: Lifespace Publishing; 1987.

31. Friedman M, Rosenman RH. Type A behavior pattern: Its association with coronary heart disease. *Am Clin Res.* 1971;3:300–312.

32. Haynes SG, Matthews KA. Review and methodologic critique of recent studies on Type A behavior and cardiovascular disease. *Ann Behav Med.* 1988;10:47–59.

33. Sotile WM. *Heart Illness and Intimacy: How Caring Relationships Aid Recovery.* Baltimore, MD: Johns Hopkins University Press; 1992.

34. Roskies E. Type A intervention: Where do we go from here? In: Strube MJ, ed. Type A Behavior. *J Soc Behav Pers.* 1990;5(special issue);419–438.

35. Parker G, Jones R. The doctor's husband. *Br J Med Psychol.* 1981;54:143–147.

36. Neser WB, Thomas J, Semenya K, Thomas J. Type A behavior and black physicians: The Meharry cohort study. *J Natl Med Assoc.* 1988;80:733–736.

37. Sterdoff B, Smith DF. Normal values for Type A behavior patterns in Danish men and women and in potential high-risk groups. *Scand J Psychol.* 1990;31:49–54.

38. Smith DF, Sterdoff B. Female physicians outscore male physicians and the general public on type A scales in Denmark. *Behav Med.* 1991–92 (Winter);17:184–189.

Stress Resilience

"The world breaks everyone. And afterward some are strong in the broken places."

Ernest Hemingway
A Farewell to Arms

We have developed certain biases from our clinical work with physicians. First, we assume that you tend to be exceptionally good at whatever you commit to doing. After all, as a group, physicians are smarter than 99% of people in the history of the world; you have an extraordinary tolerance for delaying gratification and working hard; and you tend to be more hardheaded and self-directed than any other group. In short, you have what it takes to get stuff done, when you decide to do it. Second, we assume that the best way to motivate you to change is to present conceptual frameworks that explain why changing is important and that operationalize the change process.

In this chapter, we present a number of paradigms and strategies for promoting stress resilience. We target those strategies that we have found to be the most practical and helpful in our clinical work with physicians. You are likely to find that some of these frameworks will help you to think about needed changes in your work relationships and attitudes, others will benefit your efforts to change at home. We intend for the advice we offer in this chapter to create a conceptual "toolbox" that can aid your efforts to change in virtually any arena.

LEARN WHAT RESILIENCE IS ALL ABOUT

Resilience is the ability to bounce back after being psychologically stressed. Research studies suggest that certain resilience is affected by a wide range of factors, including age, sex, social class, family dynamics, social support, temperament, self-efficacy, belief in

God, and coping skills.[1,2] Almost universally, researchers have found that individuals with higher intelligence levels are more likely to be resilient. The exact mechanism of protection here is not clear, but it is speculated that the more intelligent, the more likely one is to make self-enhancing choices. Perhaps more intelligent people are more likely to maintain an optimistic outlook, a factor that also has been found to correlate with having the sort of "sunny" disposition that temperamentally protects one from depression or neuroticism.

Having a "sunny" disposition also fosters one of the most powerful contributors to resilience: positive interactions with others. Prospective studies of children have shown that the presence of at least one supportive adult either within or outside the immediate family is crucial in promoting resilience.[1] Resilient children have also been found to actually seek out social support.[3] And research with adult populations has suggested that finding a mate who is both stable and supportive may be one way out of a troubled past.[1,4]

Clearly, some of the factors that promote resilience, like higher intelligence, are givens; they cannot be created or willed into existence. Others—like one's world view (ie, optimism versus pessimism), participation in spiritual practices, and one's interpersonal style—are amenable to being shaped by concerted effort. Wolin and Wolin[3] found that resilient individuals mindfully build on their own strengths. They deliberately and methodically work to improve the lifestyles into which they were born. And they work hard at building a cohesive family and support systems.

The flip side of resilience is also worth noting. The preeminent behavioral medicine researcher, psychiatrist Redford Williams of Duke University Medical Center, and colleagues[5] have noted that the following psychosocial, biological, and behavioral problems tend to cluster in troubled individuals:

- Hostility, depression, and social isolation
- Stress reactions mediated by overactive sympathetic nervous system
- Underactive parasympathetic nervous system calming responses
- Poor health behaviors, including poor eating habits, increased alcohol consumption, and increased cigarette smoking.

In their book, *Life-Skills*, Redford and Virginia Williams convincingly summarized the positive effects of providing patients diagnosed with cancer or heart disease with social support and/or teaching them skills to manage their negative emotions and improve their relationships. The Williamses conclude that this body of research "gives us confidence that similar interventions to help healthy people counter the forces that impair relationships will improve their health and happiness as well."[5]

In a nutshell, research in this area suggests that working to bolster resilience-promoting factors can, indeed, pay huge dividends. Doing so can attenuate the negative effects of problem factors and boost the odds of attaining reasonable levels of health and happiness.

BEGIN WITH THE END IN MIND

Wellness experts have long touted the benefits of value-based living. Our clinical experience with physicians suggests that violation of this tenet is what often fuels syndromes that lead to symptoms like irritability, anhedonia, and loss of passion about practicing medicine. Living out of harmony with one's values is akin to what happens to an automobile being driven with both the accelerator and brakes activated: burnout.

Clearly, it is important to periodically make the time to clarify your ultimate goals in life and to specify how you want to live. Some call this process "developing a personal mission statement." Doing so can take several forms.

Medical College of Pennsylvania physician Dennis Novack, MD, and colleagues[6] help resident physicians to clarify their values by posing the following questions to them: What are your priorities? Are you living your life in ways that are consistent with these priorities? If not, what are the barriers? What strategies can help accomplish these priorities?

Regularly ponder the question: Why did I enter this profession? Doing so can help clarify your value-based intentions and lead to insights regarding needed areas of behavioral change required if you are to chart a course that is true to your most deeply held values.

Exercises 4-1, 4-2, and 4-3, are simple exercises commonly used by psychotherapists, can help you to operationalize your values and develop a corresponding personal mission statement.

E X E R C I S E   4-1

Picture the End of Your Life

Imagine that, from the position of your afterlife, you are viewing your own funeral. Seven speakers address your life, someone from your immediate family, your extended family, your group of friends, your group of physician colleagues, the group of colleagues at your workplace, your group of patients, and your church or community organizations

What would you like to have said about you by each of these individuals? What personal and professional characteristics, contributions, and services would you hope to have mentioned? By writing these various aspects of your eulogy, you can clarify the values in each of these areas that you hold most dear.

E X E R C I S E   4-2

If You Only Had a Limited Time to Live

Few physicians fail to notice the wisdom that many patients demonstrate when they are faced with their own mortality. Once the shock of receiving a diagnosis of a terminal illness wears off, people often use awareness of impending death to make changes that heal their lives.

Imagine that you just learned that you have only 2 or 3 more years to live. How do you imagine you would react to this news? What would you take time to begin doing more or less of? With whom would you choose to spend your precious, remaining time? What would you be sure to do and say during this time? What aspects of your life would you look back on with pride? What would you need to forgive in yourself or others? What new experiences would you finally take the time to orchestrate? What simple pleasures would you allow yourself to mindfully enjoy on a daily basis?

DISRUPT THE DOMINOES

Our EEM counseling is based on the principle that, by recognizing the individual steps in your coping habits, you can take control of yourself at the level of "next." Your stress symptoms can be viewed as reminders to change the next step in your typical coping process. Just as with a real stack of dominoes, changing one piece changes everything thereafter. Put another way: A key to EEM is learning to disrupt overlearned coping dances by honestly answering this question: What do I typically do next and what

E X E R C I S E 4-3

I Have Finally Become the Type of Person Who. . .

Imagine that it is exactly 1 year from now. As you rummage through your bookshelves, you notice this copy of *The Resilient Physician*. You pause and realize, "I have made a number of good changes in my life during the year since I read that book. Compared to the way I used to be, I have finally become a person who. . . ." Part A of the form below is designed to help you complete this thought. In the right-hand column, specify how you would describe yourself in this self-affirming fantasy. Use the accompanying sentence starters to operationalize how you would like to be.

Part A. How I Would Like To Be

The person I've finally become:

I treat others in these ways:

I care for myself in these ways:

I tend to think about the world and other people in these ways:

I regularly make time for_____ in my life.

I've finally been able to let go of these struggles:

Answering these questions will help you to operationalize what kind of person you would *like* to become—how you would like to treat others, care for yourself, think, manage your time, and cope. The next step is to clarify how you are living *here and now* in each of these areas in Part B, noting any contrasts between how you are living and how you would like to be.

Continued on next page

E x e r c i s e   4-3   (c o n t i n u e d)

Part B. Personal Now and Future Contrasts

These days, I live like this: The person I've finally become:

I treat others in these ways: I treat others in these ways:

I care about myself like this: I care for myself in these ways:

Here's how I tend to think about the   I tend to think about the world and other
world and other people: people in these ways:

The time of my life is filled   I regularly make time for_____ in
with these activities and roles: my life.

I struggle with these issues or people: I've finally been able to let go of these
                                         struggles:

Note: The point of this exercise is to help clarify specific steps you can take that will lead to
at least small changes in each of the targeted areas. Our clinical experiences suggest that,
when it comes to becoming a better emotional manager, it is, indeed, the case that little
changes make big differences. This is very much the case when it comes to making adjustments that bring our behaviors in line with our values.

---

might I do differently *right now* to take more nurturing care of
myself in *this* situation? This does not guarantee that the new outcome will be exactly what you want. It does, however, guarantee
that you will not get lost in the same old maladaptive syndrome.
Pattern disruption gives you a chance to make something different (and, hopefully, more comfortable) happen. In the remainder
of this chapter, we offer a number of specific recommendations
about how you might shape stress-resilient next steps in your
coping process.

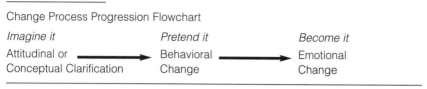

F I G U R E 4-1

Change Process Progression Flowchart

Imagine it	*Pretend it*	*Become it*
Attitudinal or Conceptual Clarification	Behavioral Change	Emotional Change

ACCEPT THE CHANGE PROCESS

Making choices that keep you in control of the pace of your life does not come naturally. In fact, when the change process is viewed in a light of honest self-appraisal, it is clear that most of the healthy choices we make lead to a feeling of awkwardness, at least in the short term. We believe that learning to bear through this awkwardness is the key to making any adaptive change. Let us elaborate.

Whether the goal is to change a maladaptive habit like temper outbursts, improve marriage and family life, or promote personal growth, the most effective change process for physicians seems to follow the progression in Figure 4-1.[7,8]

Changing is awkward. New behaviors have to be practiced until they feel familiar. We generally accept this fact when it comes to learning new skills like a new golf swing, a new medical technique, or a new dance step.

But what about when it comes to learning to be a better listener, a better lover, a more self-nurturing person, or some other personal change? Here, we often misinterpret the awkwardness that comes with practicing a new behavior. We reason that the feeling of awkwardness signals fraudulence ("If I feel this way, I must be 'faking it.'"), and we abort the change.

Reframe the awkwardness you feel as you change: You are not *faking it,* you are *practicing it.* First, *imagine* how you want to be. Clarify the change you want to make. Then commit yourself to making that change.

Next, practice *behaving* in harmony with your decision. Remember that it's okay to "pretend" to be a certain way because you have decided that's the way you want to be.

After many practice trials (pretending), your new way of acting will begin to feel natural and authentic. Only then will an emotional change occur; the imagined and pretended ways of acting start to feel natural and authentic.

COUNTER STRESS THINKING

One "behavior" that must be practiced to maintain resilience is learning to disrupt swirls of stress-generating thinking. Cognitive theorists[9] recommend that you conceptualize individual thoughts as being discrete units of "behavior" that have emotional consequences. In Chapter 1, we mentioned how important it is to manage one's attitude when coping with work stress. We now expand our focus to emphasize the importance of countering cognitive "sets" and stress-thinking patterns that diminish resilience.

Cognitions are the final common pathway that fuel our emotions. Our beliefs about ourselves and the world around us perpetuate self -statements. These private (almost always believed by us) discrete and specific messages, which usually appear in brief form, are bothersome by nature and hard to turn off. These ways of thinking create "lenses" that color our perceptions and, to a large extent, shape our physiological, behavioral, and emotional reactions. Here are a few examples of how this works.

Researcher John Gottman noted that when partners in a distressed marriage simply recall a recent argument, they have blood-pressure surges almost as high as during the actual argument.[10]

At a minimum, stress thinking results in *states* of heightened anxiety and anger. In certain circumstances, anyone may think herself into a state of anxiety or anger. But for some people, their uncomfortable emotions are not due to mere circumstances; anxiety or anger become personality *traits* rather than situation-specific *states*. Individuals who score high on measures of trait anxiety or anger tend to spread their misery to those around them.[11] For example, research in the workplace suggests that individuals with high trait anger engage in more counterproductive work behavior, such as arguing with others or sabotaging their work, than those who are not elevated on trait anger. In addition, high trait anger has been found to correlate strongly with acts against both one's work organization and other people.[12] And high trait anxiety has been found to correlate with more frequent absences from work, frustration, health symptoms, job dissatisfaction, poor well-being, and work-related anxiety.[13,14] High trait anxiety is also associated with high levels of perceived interpersonal conflict, role ambiguity, role conflict, situational constraints and skill under-utilization, and perceived low levels of autonomy.[15]

In stark contrast to the pain caused by negative thinking, researchers have documented the soothing power of engaging in loving thoughts and forgiveness. For example, try this: Think of someone you care deeply about. Vividly picture a pleasant image of that person and hold that thought or image in your mind. If you are like the subjects evaluated by Tiller and associates[16] with Holter monitoring, thinking this loving thought stirred an immediate and sustained positive effect on heart-rate variability.[16] Other researchers[17] have clearly demonstrated that learning to forgive diminishes trait anger.

A key to stress resilience is disrupting the thought patterns that come from negative beliefs about the world around us. Unfortunately, it is human nature to think in distress-generating ways when stressed. If unchecked, such broad-based beliefs are likely to lead to stress-thinking patterns like the following:

- *All-or-nothing thinking:* Seeing things in only black and white.
- *Personalizing blame:* Assuming that all that goes wrong is your fault.
- *Catastrophizing:* Imagining the worst-case scenarios.
- *Selective perception:* Scanning for negatives.

Martin[18] observed that physicians commonly manifest the following four dysfunctional belief systems: limitations in knowledge indicate a personal failing, responsibility is to be borne alone by physicians, altruistic devotion to work and denial of self is desirable, and it is "professional" to keep one's uncertainties and emotions to oneself.

Ornstein and Sobel[19] suggest that the best way to expose and get rid of negative attitudes like pessimism is to ask good questions, ones that force you to think more clearly and realistically. When you find yourself stuck in stress thinking, ask yourself some of the following questions:

- *Am I thinking in all-or-nothing terms?* Beware of words like "all," "nothing," "totally," "completely," and "forever."
- *Am I assuming every situation is the same?* Look for words like "always," "never," and "from now on."
- *Am I confusing a rare occurrence with a probability?* Ask: "When was the last time what I'm bothered by now happened in reality?"

- *Am I assuming the worst possible outcome?* Ask: "What are the odds that things will really go as badly as I am speculating they will? Even if this does happen, what would I do? Would this truly be a catastrophe? How could I turn it into an opportunity?"

- *Am I overlooking my strengths?* Ask: "What positive attributes do I possess that I am ignoring?"

- *Am I blaming myself for something that was beyond my control?* Ask: "Even though I might have chosen differently (now that I have the benefit of hindsight), did I exert at least a reasonable effort to keep this from happening?"

- *Am I expecting perfection in myself and others?* Ask: "Where did I ever get the notion that I or anyone else "should" be perfect?" Work to develop more humble self-expectations and more gracious responses to other's flaws.

- *How could I have handled this situation differently?* Other than the stress-thinking perspectives you may be engaging in, what are three alternative ways you could explain this event to yourself?

- *What difference will this make in a week, a year, or 10 years?* Ask: "Will anyone really care or judge me in the future, simply and solely based on this situation or mistake?"

In their discussion of stress-management strategies for physicians, Quill and Williamson[20] emphasized the advisability of using cognitive reframing strategies to soothe painful emotions. Here are examples of how this might be done:

- Remind yourself that death is not a villain; it sometimes is a friend that alleviates suffering.
- Remember that mistakes are opportunities to learn.
- Uncertainties come due to the nature of medical science, not due to personal limitations.
- Often, patient demands are cries for help.
- By setting limits on your availability to others, you will preserve your ability to continue to be a vibrant, caring person.

By learning to examine the internal monologue you engage in when reacting to the world, you can begin to reshape any irrational, underlying beliefs that may be shaping your responses and moods. Doing so is important because, if they are not countered with more soothing thoughts, these frames of reference compli-

---

E X E R C I S E   4-4

Life Orientation Test

Instructions: Mark how much you agree with each of the items below, using the following scale:

4 = strongly agree   3 = agree   2 = neutral   1 = disagree   0 = strongly disagree

___1. In uncertain times, I usually expect the best.

___2. If something can go wrong for me, it will.*

___3. I always look on the bright side of things.

___4. I'm always optimistic about my future.

___5. I hardly ever expect things to go my way.*

___6. Things never work out the way I want them to.*

___7. I'm a believer in the idea that "every cloud has a silver lining."

___8. I rarely count on good things happening to me.*

Scoring instructions: Reverse the numbers for the items marked with an asterisk(*). For example, if you strongly agree with the statement "I hardly ever expect things to go my way," give yourself a score of 0 instead of 4. Do this for items 2, 5, 6, and 8. Then total your score.

Total Score: ____

Interpretation: A score of 20 or above indicates that you are optimistic.
A score of 19 or below indicates that you are pessimistic.

Adapted from: Scheier MF, Carver CS. Optimism, coping, and health: Assessment and implications of generalized outcome expectancies. *Health Psychol.* 1985;4(3):219–247. Used with permission.

---

cate coping and diminish stress resilience. Work to develop cognitive habits that contribute to an optimistic point of view, even if doing so does not come naturally to you.

Optimism and Pessimism

Martin Seligman, PhD, a past-president of the American Psychological Association, has spent his career studying optimism and pessimism. His work clearly demonstrates two points. First, unchecked pessimistic thinking is dangerous. Compared to opti-

F I G U R E   4-2

Dimensions of Optimistic and Pessimistic Thinking

Stable	versus	**Unstable**
("It always happens.")		("This is a transient, one-time event.")
Global	versus	**Specific**
("I can't do anything about this.")		("This happened for a specific reason that is modifiable.")
Internal	versus	**External**
(It's all my fault.")		("Things didn't turn out so well because of circumstances that were not fully under my control.")

mists, pessimists evidence poorer health, diminished levels of well-being, and shorter life spans.[21,22] Second, Seligman[23] demonstrated that by developing the habit of countering stress thinking with cognitions that reflect a more reasonable assessment of one's circumstances and the coping options available, optimism can be learned.

You can assess your attitudinal set with the Life Orientation Test (Exercise 4-4) developed by psychologists Michael Scheier and Charles Carver.[22]

Optimistic and pessimistic thinking are differentiated based on three dimensions as seen in Figure 4-2. Research has shown that, when something goes wrong, a pessimist explains it in terms that are global, stable, and internal. ("Things will never be the same again; I can't do a thing about this; this is all my fault.") When something good happens, on the other hand, a pessimist discounts the event as unstable, specific, and external. ("The good times won't last; this won't make much difference in my life; I just had a moment of luck.")

Optimists do just the opposite of pessimists. Bad events are written off in terms that indicate unstable, specific, and external cognitions. ("Things will get better; I can learn from this experience; I just ran into a little bit of bad luck.") Optimists embrace good fortune in terms that indicate a stable, global, and internal world view. ("Now, things will be great and life will just keep getting better; my hard work paid off!")

Countering stress thinking is a lifelong endeavor but is well worth the trouble. To the extent that you fill your life with nurturing, as opposed to toxic people and processes, it will be easier to control stress thinking. We turn next to discussion of two factors that indisputably help in this endeavor: engaging in an active spiritual life and having a sense of humor.

GO TO CHURCH!

Indisputable links have been demonstrated between faith, health, and healing. Extensive reviews of this literature[24-26] concluded that 80% of published studies have demonstrated a positive relationship between religious commitment and health, regardless of ethnicity, race, socioeconomic status, gender, or age. Specifically, people who have active spiritual lives—believe in God, pray to that God, and belong to and actively participate in a faith community—are healthier and happier than those who do not. They even live longer! Compared to the nondevout, the more religiously devout drink less alcohol, smoke less, and have safer sex. They also report diminished levels of anxiety, depression, and anger compared to those who rely less on faith.

Active participation in a faith community can also benefit marriage. Couples who integrate religion into their marriage have been found to have less marital conflict, more verbal collaboration, greater marital adjustment, and more perceived benefits from marriage.[27]

Finally, people facing stressful times who report receiving significant comfort from their religious beliefs prove to be more stress resilient than those who do not. For example, in one study of coronary artery bypass patients, those who reported comfort from their religious beliefs evidenced survival at a rate that was 3 times higher than those who did not have such beliefs.[28]

It has been postulated that belief in a higher power may short-circuit nonproductive worries and doubts[29] and lead to an increased sense of inner control.[30] Spirituality and faith can also provide optimism and a secure attachment that transcends human relationships.

And least you speculate that these positive effects might be due to regional and cultural variables, these findings have been replicated with cohorts from North Carolina, New York, the Midwest, California, and Texas.[31] Sethi and Seligman[32] explored studies dating back 100 years and found that the association between religious beliefs and well-being is related to the optimism promoted by Orthodox Judaism, Calvinism, and Islamic religions.

DON'T FORGET TO LAUGH AND PLAY

One characteristic of stress-resilient people is their ability to maintain a sense of humor, despite their life's challenges. Laughter is an antidote to stress. Plus, laughing soothes one's physiology. Laughter has been shown to increase pain thresholds,[33] enhance immune system functioning,[34] and diminish stress hormones.[35] Laughter also exercises lungs, relaxes the diaphragm, increases oxygen in the bloodstream, improves mood, and activates parasympathetic calming reactions for up to 30 minutes afterward.[36]

Of course, it is difficult to maintain your sense of humor if you are living in a state of numbness. In the following pages, we discuss the importance of breaking down stress buildup by learning to focus on daily uplifts and incorporating small changes and healthy pleasures into your flow of activities. Here, we emphasize an activity that we have almost universally found physicians to be rather unfamiliar with: play.

Simply put, we develop self-efficacy for activities that we practice. Given this fact, it is understandable that many physicians are not very adept at playing. Either due to the rigors of their training and work schedules or to personality-based factors that predispose them to focus on dutiful attention to the work of their life, most physicians admit that "taking recess" is not something they have much experience doing. Add to this the propensity to turn potential "play" situations (golf, kids' activities, and so on) into work, and the odds diminish even further that "taking recess" will be a pleasurable experience.

Being playful is an effective way to connect with others, ease your own tensions, and keep perspective on yourself and the problems you face. A particular form of play unfamiliar to many high-performing people is the fine art of taking a true vacation. Physicians aren't alone in their struggle with this one. A study by the Hilton Hotel chain reported that 38% of people polled had not taken a vacation in more than a year.[37] Often, physicians develop the habit of pairing "a vacation" with attending a medical meeting. Translation: Their spouse and family are left to enjoy the resort while the physician spends all day in the bowels of a conference center, "soaking up the rays" of florescent lights!

It is wise to use your resources to take vacations. And make these vacations times of play, not times to work or to teach your children anything. This last point warrants elaboration.

Many children of physicians we counsel state that their memories of their hard-working physician parent were made on vacations, the only times they saw their parent truly relaxed and playful. Compared to making such memories, how important is it to spend your week enrolling the kids in ski school or some other competitive endeavor that carries with it the risk that your child's response to the "learning experience" will simply prove to frustrate you and further stress him or her?

In learning to enjoy vacations, it is also important to be realistic. Before leaving home, you and your mate should clarify whether you are about to take a family trip or orchestrate a romantic getaway. Any single trip is unlikely to serve both functions well. You and your mate can prevent needless disappointment and distress if you clarify your respective agendas and plan for both types of vacations: some as a family, some *sans* kids.

Also, be realistic about reentry. The relaxation and rejuvenation benefits of a vacation can quickly be erased by a work binge immediately upon returning home. Many physicians find it helpful to use one vacation day for the purpose of gradually reentering a full-fledged work schedule. Make time to catch up on mail, phone calls, and paperwork before reentering your full schedule.

DO SWEAT THE SMALL STUFF

When it comes to understanding the causes of their emotions, high-powered people typically discount the small stuff. We tend to reason, "As complicated as life gets, it couldn't make much difference to do something so fundamental or simple as _____." (Fill in the blank with a simple thing that you could do to de-stress your day in some small way.) When we abdicate responsibility for doing what is, indeed, do-able to soothe our anxieties, we feel victimized by stressors that are out of our direct control. Remember: *Managing the small stuff is the way to control yourself during uncontrollable times.*

Unfortunately, research suggests that many physicians do a poor job of attending to even the basics of self-care. For example, physicians frequently have no general practitioner of their own. Rather, most self-medicate and respond to their own illnesses by continuing to work.[38,39]

Physicians also report higher levels of sleep deprivation and fatigue than are found in the general population,[40] and they suffer for it. For example, sleep deprivation has been found to deteriorate both mood and performance.[41,42] It's no surprise that, in a recent study, the main reason given by physicians regarding why they make mistakes was tiredness.[43] Fatigue has also been found to contribute to physician anger and abuse toward patients.[43,44]

The good news is that even rudimentary stress management practices can make a tremendous, positive difference in conserving coping energies. Don't forget the basics:

- *Take advantage of any opportunity to engage in physical activity throughout the day,* even if you think that you do not have time to formally "exercise." Use the stairs, pause and walk around for a few minutes before moving on to your next task, do light stretching or calisthenics periodically between patient appointments. Even these little bouts of exercise can boost your parasympathetic calming reactions and dampen your sympathetic arousal.

- *Eat healthily.* Eating nutrient-rich meals and snacks five to six times each day has been shown to improve work efficiency, energy, and metabolism[45] and to lower blood cholesterol levels.[46] Avoid the high-stress diet of junk food, caffeine, simple sugars, and other stimulants.

- *Respect the effect your environment has on your mood.* Where possible, make these workplace adjustments that have been shown to boost productivity: increase lighting, listen to emotionally expansive background music, surround yourself with positive colors and scents.

Doing these things can enhance relaxation and increase your levels of energy, alertness, and attentiveness.[47]

We close this section with a summary of observations made by Quill and Williamson[20] who used an open-ended, two-page questionnaire that asked physicians to comment about how they take care of themselves. Their findings serve as a set of common-sense reminders.

- *Live according to your values*
  Regularly set aside time to clarify your values.
  Develop short-term and long-term goals that are realistic and related to your values.

Prioritize and develop time-management strategies that exclude low-priority commitments.

■ *Attend to scheduling*

Limit on-call and weekend work.

Schedule and take frequent vacations.

Limit evening work.

Take mini breaks during the day.

Take moments to "get ready" to see your next patient.

Protect time to be with your family or friends.

■ *Express your feelings*

Grieve your losses.

Experience joy in victories.

Laugh at your own foibles.

■ *Take care of your physical self*

Get regular sleep, meals, and time alone.

Seek regular medical and dental care.

Get regular physical stimulation (exercise, sex, massage).

■ *Regularly engage in activities that promote self-awareness*

Keep a personal journal.

Read provocative books.

Practice your religion.

Engage in continuing education outside of medicine.

Seek personal counseling or psychotherapy.

Engage in metaphysical exploration (meditation, yoga).

■ *Protect your relationships*

Protect informal time to spend with family, friends, and colleagues (discuss difficult issues, laugh over human foibles, complain, tell stories).

Participate in group interests outside of medicine (clubs, teams, courses).

Participate in experiential courses and self-awareness groups.

Use multidisciplinary health care teams.

Get help with domestic or professional tasks.

FOCUS ON DAILY UPLIFTS, NOT HASSLES

A second way to disrupt stress progressions is to engage in small spurts of pleasurable activities (uplifts) throughout the day. Uplifts are things like having positive interchanges with loved ones or friends, engaging in a pleasurable activity, contributing to something meaningful to you, or feeling good about meeting a responsibility.

Researchers have shown that daily minor irritants actually have a greater harmful impact on our health than do major life events.[48] Enjoying frequent, small pleasures, on the other hand, has been shown to have a greater effect on positive mood than do intense periods of feeling good.[49] Put another way, stress problems do not result solely from the increase in the absolute amount of *distress* in your life. Stress problems also have to do with the *absence of uplifts*, or pro-stress. Furthermore, research has shown that when you are experiencing a great deal of negative stress, incorporating uplifts in day-to-day life can help you to enjoy a higher quality of life, even though things are stressful.[50] In a nutshell, your happiness is more affected by how much time you spend feeling good on a daily basis than by momentary "peak" experiences.[49]

REGULARLY ENJOY HEALTHY PLEASURES

In their book, *Healthy Pleasures,* psychologist Robert Ornstein and physician David Sobel presented a thorough overview of research that has documented the health benefits of indulging in healthy pleasures.[19] This field of study suggests that "the healthiest people seem to be pleasure-loving, pleasure-seeking, pleasure-creating individuals."[19] The key, of course, is to engage in *healthy* pleasures. These do not include quick-fix mood changers like alcohol, binge eating, or other forms of unhealthy escapism. Rather, healthy pleasures soothe without costing us our well-being. Healthy pleasures come in many flavors. Key points from Ornstein and Sobel's[19] literature review are summarized in Table 4-1.

We recommend that you conduct a pleasure experiment. For 1 month, commit to making the time to engage in several healthy pleasures each day, even if for only brief periods of time. Try things that you might not typically do and, of course, relish doing those that you already know you enjoy.

TABLE 4-1

The Benefits of Healthy Pleasures

Activity	Effect	
	Lowers	**Enhances**
Touch	Heart rate	
Massage	Anxiety	
Sauna or hot bath	Stress hormones	Serotonin
	Pain	Beta-endorphins
		Relaxation
		Sleep
		Resistance to infection
Sunlight	Seasonal mood changes	
Viewing nature	Sadness	Alpha brain waves
		Wakeful relaxation
		Positive feelings
Pleasant sounds and music	Anxiety	Endorphins
	Pain	Relaxation
		Immune system functioning
Pleasant scents		Positive emotions
Moderate physical activity	Depression	Relaxation
	Anxiety	Parasympathetic arousal
	Stress hormones	Sleep
		Immune system functioning
		Neurochemical processing

Ornstein and Sobel recommend that you match your relaxation strategies to your tensions and preferences for stimulation. For example, if your responses to the exercise that opened this chapter suggests that you are a "body reactor" to stress, you might benefit from activities like muscle relaxation, deep breathing, walking, or hot baths.

If, on the other hand, you are a "mind reactor" to stress—that is, you react with obsessiveness, mind racing, and overfocus on bothersome thoughts—you would likely benefit from relaxation procedures that fill your consciousness with calming or benign ideation. Effective here are strategies like meditation, visualization, prayer, or imagery and activities that distract—watching television or movies, listening to music, or reading.

Ornstein and Sobel also emphasize that people vary considerably in their physiological reactions to different levels of external stimulation. For some, silence and passivity are maximally calming and rejuvenating. These are the folks who relax best when they have quiet times during which they simply keep still.

But, contrary to popular notions, this is not the *sine qua non* of healthy stress management. Many find inactivity and silence to be more agitating than soothing; they are more calmed by external stimulation that distracts or entertains. As we discuss in the following section, if you are one of these folks, the key to rejuvenating with healthy pleasures is to work periods of time that allow you to switch channels and focus on something other than your typical quest into your daily schedule.

DIVERSIFY; DON'T HUNKER DOWN

Taking brief breaks to enjoy healthy pleasures is an effective way to avoid the classic mistake of "hunkering-down," which is often done by achievement-striving professionals. This colloquialism refers to the tendency to narrow our range of focus and lock in a "wait-until" mentality, chronically delaying gratification. In our clinical offices, we hear endless variations of this theme:

"I'll wait until I finish this course before I get back to exercising regularly."

"I have to wait until I pass my boards before I can afford to take any nights off to relax."

"I'll wait until I make partner, then I'll start having a date night with my spouse."

According to the noted stress researcher Hans Selye,[51] this sort of coarctating—or narrowing one's focus of attention—actually promotes burnout and impaired performance. Specifically, by limiting the range of activities we engage in, we run the risk of depleting the coping reserves needed to adapt to the major stressors that fill our life. The result can be stress-related depression, momentary cognitive impairment, and physiological and emotional exhaustion. In prior work[52], we explained this phenomenon this way:

"Your ability to cope with stress can be thought of as depending on the availability of a precious fuel, called adaptation energy. Only a limited amount of adaptation energy is available at any point in time, and this energy is divided into "fuel tanks." Each of these tanks serves a specific purpose, depending upon your activities or stressors at the moment. Both positive and negative aspects of life can drain adaptation energy, because coping with both requires changing, and any change requires adaptation or adjustment.

Whenever you need to adapt or cope, you draw adaptation energy from the appropriate fuel tank. There are two ways that you burn off fuel from the corresponding adaptation energy channel: If you are actually dealing with a stressor related to the theme of that channel or if you are thinking about that stressor.

Stress complications occur when energy is drawn from a given channel for too long a time. When this happens, the stress response progresses from alarm to adaptation to exhaustion."[52]

According to Selye, once you enter the exhaustion stage of the stress response, bad things happen to you physically, emotionally, and cognitively. First, the bath of stress hormones that come with exhaustion can compromise or complicate your overall physical health and promote premature wear and tear on various physiological systems. A growing sense of emotional restlessness or aggravation leaves you struggling to cope and inflexible in your reactions to continued stress. Eventually, neurochemical changes that correspond with exhaustion interfere with attention, memory, and creative problem solving.

The good news is that relief from this form of exhaustion is readily available; all you have to do is regularly "switch channels." By congruently switching your focus to new activities (like enjoying healthy pleasures), you replenish your stress-managing energies. Changing your activity or focus allows the exhausted adaptation energy channel to refill its drained supply of coping energy.

"In simple terms: Damage from stress can be prevented simply by changing your activity and your focus when you notice the signals of advancing stress. In this way, energy-exhausting drain from the overused channel is stopped, and as drain from a more full adaptation energy 'tank' is started, the relatively drained tank is refueled."[52]

Research has shown that men and women who evidence a more "complex and diverse" style of living show fewer signs of stress;

less depression; and fewer incidents of foul moods, colds, stomach pains, headaches, and muscle aches.[53]

So, diversify! Even taking brief pauses in your day can help you to remain efficient and avoid exhaustion. Consider the alternative: Research has suggested that working too long at a task results in up to a 500% increase in problem-solving time.[54] Taking regular, multiple, 2-minute breaks throughout the day, on the other hand, has been shown to boost productivity and mood.[55]

FIGHT THE RIGHT FIGHT: STRIVE FOR STATES OF HIGH ENERGY/LOW TENSION

In *Executive EQ: Emotional Intelligence in Leadership and Organizations,* authors Robert K. Cooper, PhD, and Ayman Sawaf[55] summarized research that demonstrated how you feel about yourself and your work and how open you are to engaging in productive dialogue with others depend on how effectively you manage your own energy and tension levels. Specifically, the authors elaborated a four-part taxonomy originally proposed by Robert Thayer of California State University at Long Beach. As you read through the four coping paradigms suggested by this model, note the characteristics that most *appeal* to you and those that most *apply* to you (ie, those that are most descriptive of your coping style).

Tense-Tiredness (High Tension, Low Energy)

Mix fatigue with nervous tension or anxiety and you get this unpleasant mood state. Here, we drift toward pessimistic cognitive shifts; we begin to sense that life is a burden and our problems seem insurmountable. This state may be transient—like an afternoon dip in energy that is alleviated by a brief break. But if it persists to the point of having sleepless nights, depression may be triggered or indicated. According to Dr Thayer, this state creates our most undesirable moods and can lead to many variations of dysfunctional behavior, including the use of drugs and alcohol to alter mood.

Calm-Tiredness (Low Tension, Low Energy)

This pleasant state of letting go and winding down typically comes when we are comfortable, awake, and at ease, perhaps enjoying some relaxing activity. This is a relief from being focused on problems; a healthy way to wind down from the stresses of your day. Unfortunately, according to Dr Thayer, many of us rarely experience true states of calm-tiredness.

Tense-Energy (High Tension, High Energy)

This is a stress-driven state. Here, mood is characterized by high energy and an almost pleasant sense of excitement and power. Stress and strain from long hours of work leave you on "auto-pilot." You impatiently push yourself to address one task after another, rarely pausing to reflect or rest. After a while, your level of physical tension becomes imperceptible to you. This tense-energy state blunts your ability to pay attention to your own needs or those of others. It is analogous to the state of "numb-ness" that we discussed earlier.

Calm-Energy (Low Tension, High Energy)

Here, we feel serene, in control, optimistic, and peaceful. We have pleasurable body feelings and a deep sense of physical stamina and well-being. This is a state of high mental and physical reserves, a kind of "flow" state of relaxed alertness. It is a state of excellence that allows for maximal physical and emotional performance with minimal stress and struggle.

The goal implied by this conceptualization is to lessen tense-energy and tense-tiredness and promote calm-energy states. Calm-energy is the state in which we experience most positive emotions, and positive emotions can help soothe whatever ails us. Research has shown that lightheartedness, humor, and being in a good mood have marked personal, relationship, and work benefits. Positive emotions have been found to lead to more emotional openness, energy, and helpful and generous attitudes toward others and to improved work processes and judgment, such as problem solving and decision making.[56] In a nutshell, increased energy and alertness levels enable the brain and senses to be more attentive to the environment, the people in it, and to your own feelings and thoughts—necessary prerequisites to effective emotional management.

DIFFERENTIATE THE URGENT/NONURGENT AND IMPORTANT/UNIMPORTANT

Calm-energy is possible if you maintain reasonable control of the pace of your life. Noted author and consultant Steven Covey[57] recommends that you place all time-consuming activities into one of four theoretical categories by characterizing an action as being either important/unimportant or urgent/nonurgent relative to a desired goal. The four categories are:

I—Important and Urgent

II—Important and Not Urgent

III—Not Important and Urgent

IV— Not Important and Not Urgent

Within quadrant I are pressing problems, crises, deadlines, and *bona fide* emergencies. Physicians' lives tend to fill with these activities, and those who research[58] physician time management point out that physicians tend to overgeneralize this crisis management style into other areas of their life. This is a fundamental mistake. An effective lifestyle requires that you focus your energies on category II activities, those that are important but not urgent.[57]

Category II activities focus on planning, prevention, creativity, building relationships, enjoying reenergizing leisure-time activities, and maintaining increased productivity. Neglecting category II leads to a mushrooming of category I activities and a lifestyle of management by crisis. A focusing on category II, on the other hand, shrinks the amount of time spent in a crisis mentality.

Covey advises that you "steal time" from categories III and IV in order to create time for activities that are important but not urgent. This requires saying no to things that are not important to you, even if they are important to others. Category III activities are those that are unimportant to you but urgent to someone else. These activities are interruptions that leave you feeling victimized, even though someone else's needs may be getting met. Included here are activities like phone calls that may be important to someone else but that simply serve as an interruption to you; mandatory meetings with nonproductive results; and time spent satisfying the needs of others, even though doing so may not be important to your core values.

Category IV activities are considered frivolous and nonhelpful wastes of time. Included here are activities that do not rejuvenate—

watching brain-numbing television shows (as opposed to making time to enjoy a favorite program or to engage in a rejuvenating hobby), engaging in gossip (as opposed to having meaningful conversation with a trusted friend), or moving stacks of paper around a disorganized office (as opposed to getting organized). You know that you are stuck in time-wasting when you seem to be consumed by activities of the moment and find that you are having difficulty accomplishing your personal goals.

Covey cautions against leading a life that is "planless." Doing so results in continual crisis management (category I), aimless responding to the urgent agendas of others (category III), or worthless wastes of time (category IV). Rather, make choices that allow you to channel your efforts into category II—where activities are of importance but not urgent. Planning and managing your use of time allows you to eliminate time wasters and focus your energies on creating new opportunities that are in harmony with your goals and values. This sort of personal management provides balance and focus toward important goals.[58]

LEARN TO LOVE WHAT YOU HAVE TO DO

For more than two decades, psychologist Mihaly Csikszentmihalyi has studied high-performing, happy people. He conceptualizes states of excellence as *flow*—

> "the state in which people are so involved in an activity that nothing else seems to matter; the experience itself is so enjoyable that people will do it even at great cost, for the sheer sake of doing it."[59]

According to Csikszentmihalyi's research, people who regularly experience flow tend to be quite resilient, productive, and happy. Further, they tend to be intellectually curious people who love to learn things for the sake of learning; they avoid bogging into passive leisure (like watching television) and, instead, engage in active leisure-time activities that rejuvenate. Plus, they find ways to make the work of their life challenging and interesting, regardless of the form that the work takes. Here Csikszentmihalyi emphasizes the importance of learning to focus one's attention and reshape one's attitude to develop harmony between "I want" and "I must."[60] Learning to love what you have to do—be it attending to domestic chores and the routines and demands that come with child rearing, engaging in "maintenance activities" necessary to keep your marriage thriving, or addressing the end-less demands that come with practicing your profession—is a key to happiness and high-level performance.

A key to stress hardiness is to learn to do what needs to be done in your life with focused attention. According to Csikszentmihalyi, full involvement in the activities that fill our days is what makes for excellence in life. Happy, stress-hardy people pay close atten-tion to what they do every day and notice how they feel in differ-ent activities, places, times of day, and with different companions.[60] This in-the-moment awareness leads to increased joy and to cor-rections that minimize toxic stress.

DEVELOP PHILOSOPHIES THAT KEEP YOU HUMBLE AND SELF-OBSERVING

As discussed in Chapter 1, physicians are not taught to suffer mistakes kindly. Stress-resilient physicians learn to accept that certain negative stressors—including unwanted medical out-comes, disappointing choices made by other family members, and frustrations in their own career progression—will inevitably occur and be accompanied by vulnerable feelings that must be dealt with in adaptive ways.

At such times, avoid the classic syndrome evidenced by many high-performing people when they are momentarily stripped of control: Waves of anxiety and shame lead to defensive reactions and focusing on how others enrage and disappoint you. Subsequent anger leads to sullen withdrawal, uncooperative silence, and attacks directed at convenient targets—all as a means of diverting your attention from your own pain.

Learning to endure disappointment and frustration without engaging in other or self-destructive behavior is, indeed, a hall-mark characteristic of resilient individuals. Perhaps it will help to remind yourself that fully 50% of people in executive positions fail at some time in their careers.[61] Quill and Williamson[20] encour-aged physicians to work to develop the view that vulnerable feel-ings are powerful resources rather than weakness to be overcome. Further, these researchers reported that stress-resilient physicians tend to be more personally nurturing and to counter unhealthy behavior patterns and feelings of isolation or depression by see-ing them as signals of a need for support or change. Resist the temptation to use coping strategies that leave you feeling victimized.

Remember that coping flexibility is the key to stress hardiness. Such flexibility requires keeping perspective on the problems that face you; honestly observing your own attitudes, emotions, and behaviors; and being able to proactively pursue adaptive coping choices.

BE GENEROUS AND BE GRACIOUS

"Afterwards I always feel calm but energized. It gives me a warm glowing feeling. An almost physical sensation in my chest."

"I was hesitant at first, but now I can hardly live without it. It's what gives my life meaning."

"I find it relieves my arthritis pain better than any medication."

"It gives me a chance to forget myself."

No, these comments do not refer to the afterglow of satisfying sexual experiences (the option most often offered when we ask participants in our workshops on physician renewal "What's your guess as to what these statements are referring to?"). In truth, these are the comments of hospital volunteers describing their feelings about helping others.[62] Helping others with acts of unselfish kindness has been shown to not only lead to positive feelings but to positive health effects. In the famous 10-year study of 2,700 residents in Tecumseh, Michigan,[63] males who reported regular involvement in volunteerism had death rates 2½ times lower than those men who did not volunteer. In fact, the investigators concluded "doing volunteer work, more than any other activity, dramatically increased life expectancy and probably health as well."[26] In a more recent study of 1,972 elderly people in California, *any* amount of volunteering lessened mortality by 60%.[64]

In *The Medical Marriage,* we observed that physicians and their families often remind us of modern-day heroes.[8] Here we are not referring to those who perform extraordinary acts. Rather, we define a hero as someone who creates safe spaces for other people. How? With acts of generosity and graciousness.

Be Generous and Be Gracious.

No message we know of can better ensure stress hardiness. Generously offer to other people the kind of attention, support, conversation, and respect that *they* need in order to feel safe in your presence. And graciously respond to such "gifts" offered you by others. In so doing, you will, at minimum, regularly create moments of caring connection of the sort that will ensure two things: You will be a source of stress hardiness for others and, in the process of creating this caring connection, your own levels of stress hardiness will be boosted.

CONCLUSIONS

We close with a reminder that, regardless of your self-management strategies, life will remain stressful. This is a simple statement of fact.

But here's the good news: There is no tragedy in having a stressful life. The only tragedy is failing to enjoy the life you have. Doing so requires that you develop a realistic, effective way to deal with the ever-present life/work juggling act. We turn next to discussion of this crucial aspect of stress resilience.

REFERENCES—CHAPTER 4

1. Werner EE, Smith RS. *Overcoming the Odds.* Ithaca, NY: Cornell University Press; 1992.

2. Garmezy N, Masten AS. Stress, competence, and resilience: Common frontiers for therapist and psychopathologist. *Behav Ther.* 1986;17:500–521.

3. Wolin SJ, Wolin S. *The Resilient Self: How Survivors of Troubled Families Rise Above Adversity.* New York, NY: Ullard Books; 1993.

4. Vaillant GE. *The Wisdom of the Ego.* Cambridge, Mass: Harvard University Press; 1993.

5. Williams R, Williams V. *Life-Skills.* New York, NY: Times Books; 1997.

6. Novack DH, Kaplan C, Epstein RM, Clark W, et al. Personal awareness and professional growth: A proposed curriculum. *Med Encounter.* 1997;13:2–8.

7. Sotile WM, Sotile MO. *Beat Stress Together: The BEST Way to a Passionate Marriage, a Healthy Family, and a Productive Life.* New York, NY: John Wiley & Sons; 1999.

8. Sotile WM, Sotile MO. *The Medical Marriage: Sustaining Healthy Relationships for Physicians and Their Families.* Chicago, Ill: American Medical Association; 2000.

9. Burns D. *Feeling Good: The New Mood Therapy.* New York, NY: New American Library; 1980.

10. Gottman J, Silver N. *Why Marriages Succeed or Fail.* New York, NY: Simon and Schuster; 1994.

11. Spielberger CD, Krasner SS, Solomon EP. The experience, expression and control of anger. In Janisse MP, ed. *Health Psychology: Individual Differences and Stress.* New York, NY: Springer; 1988:89–108.

12. Spector PE. Individual differences in the job stress process of health care professionals In: Firth-Cozens J, Payne R, eds. *Stress in Health Professionals: Psychological and Organisational Causes and Interventions.* New York, NY: John Wiley & Sons; 1999:33–42.

13. Jex SM, Spector PE. The impact of negative affectivity on stressor-strain relationships: A replication and extension. *Work and Stress.* 1996;10:36–45.

14. Moyle P. The role of negative affectivity in the stress process: Tests of alternative models. *J Organ Behav.* 1995;16:647–668.

15. Chen PY, Spector PE. Negative affectivity as the underlying cause of correlations between stressors and strains. *J Appl Psychol.* 1991;76:398–407.

16. Tiller W, McCraty R, Atkinson M. Cardiac coherence: A review of non-invasive measure of autonomic nervous system order. *Alter Ther Health Med.* 1996;2(1):52–65.

17. Coyle CT, Renright RD. Forgiveness intervention with postabortion men. *J Clin Comm Psychol.* 1997;65:1042–1046.

18. Martin AR. Stress in residency: A challenge of personal growth. *J Gen Intern Med.* 1986;1:252–257.

19. Ornstein R, Sobel D. *Healthy Pleasures.* Reading, Mass: Addison-Wesley Publishing Co; 1989.

20. Quill DE, Williamson PR. Healthy approaches to physician stress. *Arch Intern Med.* 1990;150:1857–1861.

21. Mossey JM, Shapiro E. Self-rated health: A predictor of mortality among the elderly. *Am J Public Health.* 1982;72:800–807.

22. Scheier MF, Carver CS. Optimism, coping, and health: Assessment and implications of generalized outcome expectancies. *Health Psychol.* 1985;4(3):219–247.

23. Seligman MEP. *Learned Optimism.* New York, NY: Alfred A. Knopf; 1991.

24. Matthews DA, Larson DB, Barry CP. *The Faith Factor: An Annotated Bibliography of Clinical Research on Spiritual Subjects.* Rockville, Md: John Templeton Foundation, National Institute for Healthcare Research; 1994.

25. Luskin F. Review of the effect of spiritual and religious factors on mortality and morbidity with a focus on cardiovascular and pulmonary disease. *IJ Cardiopulmonary Rehabil.* 2000;20:8.

26. Levin JS. Religion and health: Is there an association, and is it casual? *Soc Sci Med.* 1994;38:1475–1482.

27. Mahoney A, Pargament TJ, Swank AB, Scott E, Emery E, Rye M. Marriage and the spiritual realm: The role of proximal and distal religious constructs in marital functioning. *J Fam Psychol.* 1999; 13:321–338.

28. Oxman TE, Freeman DH Jr, Manheimer ED. Lack of social participation or religious strength and comfort as risk factors for death after cardiac surgery in the elderly. *Psychosom Med.* 1995;57:5–15.

29. Benson H, Stark M. *Timeless Healing: The Power and Biology of Belief.* New York, NY: Scribner; 1996.

30. Justice B. *Who Gets Sick: How Beliefs, Moods, and Thoughts Affect Your Health.* Los Angeles, CA: Tarcher; 1988.

31. Koenig H. Faith/Healing. *The Winston Salem Journal,* May 2, 1998, p. D-1.

32. Sethi S, Seligman MEP. Optimism and fundamentalism. *Psychol Sci.* 1993;4:256–269.

33. Cogan R, Cogan D, Waltz W, McCue M. Effects of laughter and relaxation on discomfort thresholds. *Int J Behav Med.* 1987;10(2):139–144.

34. Dillon KM, Minchoff B, Baker Kh. Positive emotional states and enhancement of the immune system. *Int J Psychiatry in Med.* 1985–86; 15:13–17.

35. Berk LS, Tan SA, Nehlsen-Cannarella SL, Napier BJ, et al. Laughter decreases cortisol, epinephrine, and 3,4-dihydroxyphenyl acetic acid (DOPAC) [abstract]. Society of Behavioral Medicine; 1988.

36. Ravicz S. *High on Stress: A Woman's Guide to Optimizing the Stress in Her Life.* Oakland, Calif: New Harbinger Press; 1998.

37. Reinhold BB. *Toxic Work.* New York, NY: Dutton, 1996.

38. Baldwin PJ, Dodd M, Wrate RW. Young doctors' health—I. How do working conditions affect attitudes, health and performance? *Soc Sci Med.* 1997;45:35–40.

39. Pullen D, Lonie CE, Lyle DM, Cam DE, Doughty MV. The medical care of doctors. *Med J Aust.* 1995; 162:481–484.

40. Hardy G, Shapiro DA, Borrill CS. Fatigue in the workforce of National Health Service Trusts; symptomatology and links with minor psychiatric disorder, demographic, occupational and work roles factors. *J Psychosom Res.* 1997;43:83–92.

41. Firth-Cozens J. Stress, psychological problems, and clinical performance. In: Vincent C, Ennis M, Audley RMJ, eds. *Medical Accidents.* Oxford: Oxford University Press; 1993.

42. Deary IJ, Tait R. Effects of sleep disruption on cognitive performance and mood in medical house officers. *BMJ.* 1987;295:1513–1516.

43. Firth-Cozens J, Greenhalgh J. Doctors' perceptions of the links between stress and lowered clinical care. *Soc Sci Med.* 1997;44:1017–1022.

44. McKee M, Black N. Does the current use of junior doctors in the United Kingdom affect the quality of medical care? *Soc Sci Med.* 1992;34:549–558.

45. Jenkins DA, et al. Nibbling versus gorging: Metabolic advantages of increased meal frequency. *N Engl J Med.* 1989;321:929–934.

46. Edelstein SL, et al. Increased meal frequency associated with decreased cholesterol concentrations. *Am J Clin Nutr.* 1992;55:664–669.

47. Gallagher W. *The Power of Place: How Our Surroundings Shape Our Thoughts, Emotions, and Actions.* New York, NY: Poseidon; 1993.

48. Kanner AD, Coyne JC, Shaefer C, Lazarus RS. Comparison of two modes of stress measurement: Daily hassles and uplifts versus major life events. *J Behav Med.* 1981;4:1–39.

49. Larsen RJ, Diener E, Cropanzano RS. Cognitive operations associated with individual differences in affect intensity. *J Pers Soc Psychol.* 1987;53:767–774.

50. Reich JW, Zatura A. Life events and personal causation: Some relationships with satisfaction and distress. *J Pers Soc Psychol.* 1981;41:1002–1012.

51. Selye H. *The Stress of Life.* New York, NY: McGraw-Hill; 1976.

52. Sotile WM. *Psychosocial Interventions for Cardiopulmonary Patients: A Guide for Health Professionals.* Champaign, Ill: Human Kinetics; 1996.

53. Linville PW. Self-complexity as a cognitive buffer against stress-related illness and depression. *J Pers Soc Psychol.* 1987;52:663–676.

54. Norfolk, D. *Executive Stress.* New York, NY: Warner; 1986

55. Cooper RK, Sawaf A. *Executive EQ: Emotional Intelligence in Leadership and Organizations.* New York, NY: Grosset/Putnam; 1997.

56. Isen AM, et al. The influence of positive affect on the unusualness of word associations. *J Pers Soc Psychol.* 1985;48:1413–1426.

57. Covey S. *The Seven Habits of Highly Effective People.* New York, NY: Simon & Schuster; 1989.

58. Brunicardi FC, Hobson FL. Time management: A review for physicians. *J Natl Med Assoc.* 1996; 88:581–587.

59. Csikszentmihalyi M. *Flow: The Psychology of Optimal Experience.* New York, NY: Harper Perennial; 1990.

60. Csikszentmihalyi M. *Finding Flow: The Psychology of Engagement with Everyday Life.* New York, NY: Basic Books; 1997.

61. Hogan R, Curphy GJ, Hogan J. What we know about leadership: Effectiveness and personality. *Am Psychol.* 1994;49:493–504.

62. Luks A. Helpers' high. *Psychol Today.* 1988; 22:39–42.

63. House JS, Robbins C, Metzner HL. The association of social relationships and activities with mortality. *Amer J Epidemiol.* 1982;116:123-140.

64. Oman D, Thoresen CE, McMahon K. Volunteerism and mortality among the community-dwelling elderly. *J Health Psychol.* 1999;4:301–316.

The Balancing Act

"A hero is someone who creates safe spaces for other people."

Wayne and Mary Sotile
The Medical Marriage[1]

How can a busy physician or couple negotiate appropriate balance between work, family, and personal needs? This is arguably one of the most daunting questions facing physicians today. Answering this question is so important that we devoted an entire book to the topic. In this chapter, not only do we summarize the advice offered in *The Medical Marriage*,[1] we also report new concepts and research findings that relate to how physicians and their loved ones, from all walks of life—not only those who are married—can stay loving sources of stress hardiness for each other.

WORK–LIFE BALANCE: AN ISSUE FOR ALL PHYSICIANS

The "road maps" that prior generations of physicians and medical families used to determine what they needed to do in order to be successful at home and at work are generally outdated. Ours is a new day, and creative institutions, hospitals, medical practices, couples, and families of all forms are recognizing both the complexities and importance of attending to work–life issues.

The greater than 85% of physicians who marry at some time[2] are the most frequent targets of this discussion. However, we emphasize that work–life balance is not solely the concern of people in traditional marriages. Single individuals also face the challenge of satisfying their work, family, and personal needs. In addition, the more than 11 million Americans currently living with unmarried partners[3] face challenges to work–family balance that are quite similar to those experienced by traditional families.

In this latter regard, Marshall Miller and Dorian Solot,
founders of the Alternatives to Marriage Project, pointed out just
how diverse today's "families" are:

"We have unmarried couples, singles not in relationships, divorced people,
stepfamilies, gay and lesbian couples who can't legally marry, people who
live together with and without children. We need to recognize and validate all
kinds of families and to support… policies that recognize all kinds, not only
married couples."[3]

No definitive statistics regarding the living arrangements or sexual orientation of today's physicians or medical trainees exist.
However, when it comes to resilience, this may be a moot point.
"It's not family form but the quality of relationships that matters
most for hardiness."[4] This statement by Froma Walsh, PhD, the
preeminent University of Chicago family researcher, reminds us
that, regardless of the structure of a relationship, it's how the
players treat each other that affects their stress resilience. Further,
it is clear that every relationship faces its own unique challenges.

Dr Walsh's cautioning is supported by a wealth of research[5,6]
suggesting that supportive family relationships are crucial to
adaptive coping. Specifically, how intimate partners treat each
other has been found to be one of the most powerful determinants of individual mental and physical well-being and work
productivity. And robust correlations exist between job satisfaction, health, happiness, and quality of marriage and family life.[7,8]
Stress in one role "bleeds" into other roles,[6] but harmony at home
seems to bolster one's ability to cope with life's total package.
Summarizing research in this area, Williams and Williams[9]
concluded that:

"Aside from high self-esteem, marital happiness contributes more to a person's
happiness than anything else, including work and friendships. On the other hand,
persistent problems within marriages are associated with increased distress, and
unmarried people are happier on average than those in troubled marriages."[9]

In our 23 years of practice, we have had the privilege of treating
more than 700 physicians. These experiences have given us private
glimpses into the many ways that physicians have addressed the
challenge of lifestyle balance. We have found that, independent of
the form of their personal relationships, successful physicians distinguish themselves in clear ways from comrades who are less for-
tunate. Key lessons we have learned from these heroic physicians

and their loved ones about how to face the challenge of juggling multiple roles fill the pages that follow. We begin by challenging a popular notion. We call it the myth of the balanced life.[10]

GIVE UP THE MYTH OF THE BALANCED LIFE

In her commencement address to the 1999 graduating class of Villanova University, novelist Anna Quindlen cautioned, "Don't ever confuse the two, your life and your work. The second is only part of the first."

This advice resonates intuitively with most of us. But this is also true: Virtually no one lives a "balanced" life. In fact, this mythical balance is today's version of the Beaver Cleaver family myth. It is an unrealistic yardstick that serves to demoralize those who use it to evaluate themselves.[10] Research supports our contention that no one lives in perfect balance between work, family, marriage, and self-focused pursuits. For example, in a recent survey of 21,501 married couples from 50 states,[11] 82% of couples reported having the problem, "I wish my partner had more time and energy for recreation with me."

We even misconstrue the term balance.

> "Remember that balance is dynamic, not a static process. The key is to repeatedly and regularly readjust your efforts and attend to the arenas of your life that have been relatively neglected in the immediate past."[10]

Unfortunately, we have created a "new-age guilt" that invites us to restrain our joy and excitement and feel bad about the time we put into our jobs. *It's okay to love your work!* In fact, the happiest and healthiest people tend to have high levels of passion, both for their loved ones and for their work.[12] Stress-hardy individuals and couples inevitably go through periods of overfocusing on one aspect of life or another (work, family, marriage, self). The key is that they do not lock in the "wait-until" mentality and let the various important aspects of their lives atrophy from *chronic* lack of attention. The antidote to the "wait-until" lifestyle is to regularly create at least moments of appropriate self-care and at least brief periods of caring connection with loved ones, especially during the busy stretches. Remember, when it comes to improving the quality of your relationships, little changes yield powerfully positive differences. Thriving individuals and couples do, indeed, tend to live busy lives. But along the way, they follow a few guidelines that are worth emulating:

- Never turn a monthly calendar without blocking out a 12- to 48-hour period of time that you designate as "relationship time." Protect that commitment just as you would your on-call schedule or your commitment to take your child to his orthodontist appointment. *And show up with your teeth brushed and your hair combed!* Most couples lose their romance out of neglect, not lack of love.

- Each day, find time to have multiple, brief, nurturing interactions with people who matter to you. Psychologist Peter Frankel reminds us that there are many ways to tell another person "I love you" (if appropriate) or "I appreciate you" or "I admire you" or "I miss you" that take less than 20 seconds.[13] Throughout each day, regularly take 20-second breaks to make contact. Try doing this for a total of 10 minutes every day. It can help you to stay connected, even during the difficult times.

- Learn to say no. "Every time someone asks you to do something, you are entering a negotiation that requires you to give up some of your time if you say yes."[14] Before agreeing to requests, consider the following questions:

  How much will be involved?

  Will the work have to be done at home and at night?

  Will I have to give up or postpone more important or lucrative work in order to accomplish the tasks involved?

  Do I really have the time to do this project?

  Will I have to give up family time or much-needed recreation or vacation time to complete the task?

  Do I really want to do this project?

We also recommend that, when possible, you limit on-call, weekend, and evening work. Set reasonable limits on the extent to which you are available to patients and colleagues. Contrary to mythology that may drive your own and other's expectations, a good physician is *not* at the beck and call of anyone who wants anything from him or her at any time. Managing yourself for the long haul requires that you learn to say no. Babitsky and Mangraviti[14] listed various polite ways to do so when dealing with requests for your time:

- "I would love to, but my plate is full."
- "That sounds great, but I'm swamped."

- "I am honored, but I'm now focusing on other areas."
- "I'm sorry, but that's out of the question. I've been out of the office and I'm just trying to dig out here."

Saying no to patient requests can also be done with compassion but clarity:

- "I am so sorry that you're having difficulty. I'm not available, but someone I know and trust is. Please let me refer you."
- "I'm really concerned about you. I'm sorry that I don't have more time today to discuss this. Would you consider scheduling a follow-up appointment, just for us to sit down and explore this further?"
- To a nurse or assistant: "Please let Mr X know that I am concerned and that I'm sorry I could not return his call personally. But I recommend that he do the following. . .."

In *Beat Stress Together*, we pointed out that saying no also involves taking charge of your lifestyle. This can be done by scheduling unplanned days. We recommend that you set aside at least one day each month that is proclaimed an unplanned day. You might find that, at first, such days fill with anxiety. But experience will teach you to enjoy meandering—one of the best ways to rejuvenate otherwise exhausted channels of energy.

Consider taking many, mini-vacations. If you want to manage stress, keep your family relationships healthy, and maintain reasonable work–life balance, there is no doubt that taking multiple, brief vacations each year is far more effective than "saving up" to take only a few, lengthy breaks. In this regard, we routinely recommend that if, for example, you allocate 20 days per year for vacation, it is most effective to plan seven, 2-day mini-vacations into the mix. Think small.

Small doses of self-nurturing can help to keep you stress resilient. Remember our aforementioned comments about the restorative value of engaging in healthy pleasures and dare to take time for pleasure, not productivity.

"Take a nap. Read something for its entertainment value. . .Take a walk. . .that is *not* according to your exercise schedule. Remember, there are 336 half-hour stretches of time in each week. You can afford to simply enjoy some of them— alone and together—and many more will remain for completing your work."[10]

Trust yourself. We have noted that many high-performing people seem frightened of their ability to rebel. They seem to fear that if they start to relax and play a bit, they'll completely drop out. In truth, regularly taking time out simply leads to more happiness and motivation, not to rebellion or sloth.

Use a join-your-family beeper. We regularly let the beepers of our age disconnect us from each other. Whether from phone calls, faxes, pagers, express mail, we allow the requests of others to invade our lives. Waters and Saunders[15] posed the intriguing question: "What would happen if you had a beeper that regularly sounded the alarm to join your family?"

Finally, Brunicardi and Hobson[16] point out that time management strategies for physicians require planning in advance, setting goals, establishing priorities, delegating responsibilities, and minimizing procrastination and interruptions (these last two are the major obstacles that keep most people from achieving well-established goals). The authors recommend that you use time logs to help evaluate and plan your long-range goals, your daily activities related to these goals, and time robbers that tend to keep you from accomplishing desired tasks.

RECOGNIZE THAT, FOR TODAY'S PHYSICIANS, FAMILY MATTERS

In the year 2000, *Medical Economics* surveyed 10,000 randomly selected physicians about details of their personal lives. A total of 2,008 physicians from all major fields in every part of the country responded (1,603 males, 386 females, 19 of unspecified gender).[17] Comparison of the survey results with a similar survey conducted in 1979 sheds light on how medical marriages have changed over the past two decades. Consider:

- *Medical marriages do last.* On average, survey respondents were married for 20 years. In 1979, the percentage of women physicians divorced or separated was 6 times higher than that of male physicians. In 2000, the ratio was only 2 to 1. An astounding 93% of physicians in the 2000 survey rated their marriages as terrific or good.

- *Physicians want a partnership.* Physicians rated mutual respect, children, and having similar interests tops on their list of factors that strengthen marriage. Seventy-five percent of physicians stated that they were satisfied with their sex life. And in 2000 there were half as many physician adulterers as in 1979.

- *Balance is important.* Compared to 1979 data, twice as many physicians today (45%) complained "I am not home enough."

This survey does not represent a controlled study of medical marriages. Only 19% of the survey respondents were women and only one member of a couple was interviewed (personal communication with Robert Lowes, January 2001). But the fact remains that this sample of 2,000 physicians reported extraordinarily high levels of marital–family satisfaction and a commitment to maintaining family health, a finding that certainly matches our impressions gleaned from decades of consulting with and counseling medical families.

BEWARE THE SUPERCOUPLE SYNDROME

For busy people, "take good care of yourself" is far easier said than done. The high-demand, low-control stressors that fill most homes and workplaces today can compel anyone to begin coping in high-powered, Type A ways. When high-performing people marry each other (which they typically do!), they tend to develop coping habits that serve them well in managing their busy lives but that may hurt their relationships. We call this the supercouple syndrome:[10] When your coping style drains your tolerance, passion, and joy, your relationships lose their zest, your family loses its warmth, and your creativity dwindles.

Supercouple syndrome results from misapplication of those wonderfully adaptive coping skills like multitasking (doing and thinking multiple things at once), being goal directed and efficient; hypervigilance (scanning for flaws and correcting them), delaying gratification, and staying focused on work and achievements. All of these are positive and necessary ways of coping. . . sometimes. But our relationships suffer when we overuse these tools. Remember: *What makes us successful at work does not necessarily make us successful at home.*

Our advice: Do your family a favor. Someplace between where you park your car and enter your home, place a reminder—"No superpeople live here."[10] Remember that of all the people in the history of the world, the handful that are *the most important people in your life today* are in the building you are about to enter. Be mindful. Bless them, don't stress them, with your presence.

ACCEPT THAT YOU ARE PART OF A SYSTEM

You cannot expect your relationships to feel any better than you do. When we flash this simple reminder onto the screen during our lectures to physicians, heads start nodding throughout the audience. Like many high-achieving people, physicians tend to fill their days with self-denial and then arrive home each evening in a marked state of emotional and physical depletion. Often, there is the explicit or implicit expectation that the family will nurture, stimulate, or otherwise entertain the exhausted one back to life. But, given that emotions are contagious, what happens next is predictable: The exhausted family member actually "drains the life" out of the family.

This is even more pronounced if the exhausted person is male. Research supports our clinical observation. Burnout experts Jackson and Maslach[18] compared husbands' job-related affective well-being with their wives' descriptions of at-home behavior. The level of husbands' job-related emotional exhaustion was significantly associated with wives reporting that

1. the husband came home tense, unhappy, tired, and upset;
2. the husband had difficulty sleeping at night; and
3. the husband's job-related difficulties contributed to a low quality of family life.

Similarly, a recent study of two-income families dispelled the myth that "If Mama's not happy, nobody's happy." Larson and Richards[19] found that, in fact, the father's mood has a more pronounced, definitive effect on the moods of the rest of the family than does the mood of any other family member.

Never underestimate the impact you have on each other. How you treat each other creates an interpersonal environment that either stresses or soothes you. The consequences are noteworthy. Research with physician samples has clearly shown that the greater the support from loved ones, the lower the role strain and the greater the overall life satisfaction.[20]

To fine-tune your connections with your loved ones, we recommend that you regularly take the "catastrophe" test, which we discuss more fully in our chapter on coping with change (Chapter 11). In a nutshell, we recommend that each day as you return home, let some landmark that you always pass (like a stop light, road sign, or intersection) cue this fantasy: "Suppose that when I get home, my mate tells me 'I no longer love you; I love someone else.' I would beg him or her to give me a second chance if I did more or less of what?" This simple fantasy can serve to remind you to attend to the small things that make big differences in keeping your caring connection alive.

USE YOUR RESOURCES AND RESOURCEFUL-NESS TO BOLSTER YOUR SUPPORT SYSTEMS

Caring for yourself and bolstering your support systems go hand in hand. Crucial to EEM is learning to appropriately self-nurture and surround yourself with supportive people, those who offer a combination of tangible support (ie, they help you to get the "stuff" of your life done), emotional support (ie, they bolster and encourage you), and informational support (ie, they help you obtain the information and services you need in order to manage your life).

To truly calm your coping style requires that you de-stress your environment and your role demands as best you can. A number of worthwhile tips on ways to do so have come from physicians themselves. A 1992 national survey asked how women in academic medicine balanced career and family responsibilities.[21] Four hundred thirty women physicians working full time in academic medicine responded. All respondents were under the age of 50 (mean age 38 years) and 63% were mothers. The 1,117 strategies suggested in this study and others[22] can be grouped into general categories that serve as good advice for any physician, male or female.

Change Structural Aspects of Your Personal and Professional Lives Where Possible

If possible do the following:

- Hire help at work and/or home. For example, you might purchase domestic support (eg, a house cleaner, yard help, dry cleaners who deliver and pick up, or an accountant to handle monthly bills).

- Strive for geographic proximity that de-stresses your life. For example, you might choose to live within easy access to your work, day care, schools, dry cleaners, grocery stores, and so forth.
- Limit certain personal/social activities, like entertaining, in order to create more time to relax.
- Limit and restructure your professional activities. Where possible, end your work days at designated times unless there are emergencies; limit academic "extras" such as committee work; and delegate or negotiate tasks that do not need to be done by you.

Change Your Personal Expectations

A notion often bantered about in psychology circles (and generally attributed to William James) holds that self-worth is a function of achievements over expectations. If this is the case, what a bane to well-being is perfectionism! Having a reasonably balanced life may require scaling down perfectionistic aspirations, within both your personal and professional lives. Respondents in the Levinson et al[21] survey clearly indicated that, in the trenches of real life, compromises must be made and tolerated. Accepting the discomfort that comes with saying no to your own vision of excellence can be difficult, but is an essential part of managing your lifestyle.

- Don't be confused by or inappropriately give into the feelings of vague anxiety that come as you make appropriate self-caring choices.[1,10] Make time for spiritual, emotional, and physical renewal and bear through any awkwardness or feeling of "playing hooky" as you take time to engage in these activities.
- To the extent you can, partition and separate your roles so that you can leave the world of home behind when you go to work and you can leave the world of work behind you when you go home.
- Change your standards to make your life more user-friendly, both at work and at home. Learn to change or to ignore unnecessary pressures to have a perfectly clean and decorated home, a perfectly tuned body, or other super-achiever quests. Regularly participate in family activities and take family

vacations that are truly vacations, not just "add-ons" to professional meetings.

- Eliminate some roles entirely. Here, make choices in harmony with your values. Are you willing to make the career and personal sacrifices that will be required if you have children? Is the extra money, prestige, and notoriety that certain professional activities bring really worth the effort required? Reevaluate every few months and change something if it's not working.

Increase Your Efficiency

Consider whether taking the time to learn certain skills might save you time and aggravation in the long run.

- Consider learning to speed read, use a day planner, update your computer skills, or take a cooking class that teaches easy ways to prepare quick meals.
- Spend brief periods of time each day getting organized, both at home and work. Doing so can ultimately save you time as you move through your busy days.

Self-Nurture

Take advantage of opportunities to self-nurture. Don't forget to enjoy the "sweet" aspect of bittersweet experiences.

- Even though you may not like having to be away from your family in order to fulfill career obligations that require you to travel, find ways to take advantage of the break. Rather than exhaust yourself with overwork or guilt about being away from home, allow the trip to rejuvenate you. Enjoy room service. Treat yourself to a massage at the hotel spa. Relax and watch a movie.
- Don't spend every minute on a business trip working. If you do, you will give your family the double-stress of not only having to tolerate your being away but then having to suffer the effect when you return home exhausted and more stressed than ever. Take care of yourself so that you can arrive home at least somewhat rejuvenated, and your loved ones, too, will benefit from your trip.

Be Realistic

Always have backup plans. Family emergencies do happen, and you need to accept this fact. Also keep in mind that the best-laid family contingency plans are made to be changed. Remember: "Although organization is important, flexibility is essential."[23]

Choose a Goal-Compatible Partner

Choose a partner who shares your goals or change your goals. Speaking of the plight of women physicians, Carnes[22] cautioned: "If a woman's goal is to be a tenured professor and her spouse's goal is to marry a domestic goddess, the relationship is doomed to fail."

Be Fair

A soul-splitting dilemma stresses many medical families: *Both* mates in most marriages today are high-performing individuals who value *both* their work and their family. Furthermore, regardless of how consciousness-raised a couple may be regarding their rights and desires for an egalitarian relationship, in the trenches of day-to-day life, someone inevitably assumes the role of being the primary caretaker of home and hearth. In most marriages, even those consisting of two physicians, that person is the wife.[24]

Results from the aforementioned survey of 21,501 married couples[11] suggest that how you go about managing your division of roles can have marked effects on your marital happiness. Specifically, within their broad sample, the researchers compared 5,153 couples where both partners indicated on a standardized marital inventory that they were happily married, with 5,127 couples where both partners reported an unhappy marriage. The researchers noted that couples who perceived their relationship as traditional in terms of roles *were much more likely to be unhappy* than couples who perceived their relationship as equalitarian. Specifically, more than four fifths of the couples in which both spouses perceived their relationship as traditional reported unhappy marriages, while less than one-fifth reported being happy. Similarly, when both people perceived their relationship as equalitarian, more than four-fifths rated their marriage as happy, while less than one-fifth were unhappy.

This is a complex and controversial finding but one that cannot be ignored, given the size of the sample. We have noted that the actual division of responsibilities has less to do with the quality of marriage than does the extent to which there exists reciprocal appreciation for each partner's contributions.

> "You must work to maintain equity: The sum total of what each of you contributes to your life together needs to be roughly equivalent in value. And perhaps more importantly, each of you needs to *make note* of what the other gives and *regularly express appreciation* for all that your partner contributes to your life together."[1]

An interesting footnote is worthy of mention here. Research suggests that, compared to their wives' estimates of their degree of involvement in domestic chores, men tend to overestimate their involvement and women to underestimate their husbands' involvement in domestic chores.[25]

This is an intriguing and challenging finding, given the results of a study that highlights some of the relationship consequences of role divisions in medical marriages. Landau et al[26] studied 108 residents and fellows in internal medicine (Seventy-two percent were male; 54% were single; 44% were married; 17% lived with a significant other; and most partners or spouses [61%] were either physicians or health care personnel. Only two partners were housewives or not working.).

If the spouse of a resident performed chores alone, there was a higher level of relationship stress. Even though spouses tended to work more than 40 hours a week, 51% of the male residents reported that their spouses or partners did the chores alone. Only 15% of the female residents' spouses did the chores alone. The authors concluded that "Male physicians who conform to sex-role stereotyping that limits their involvement in chores and family life may, therefore, create marital discord."[26]

A final note about this issue. Six out of 10 women say that more support from their husbands is the single biggest factor that would help them balance work and family responsibilities.[10] And cutting-edge research has documented that work–family balance is a two-sided coin. Researcher Michael r Frone of the State University of New York analyzed data from 2,700 men and women who were employed and either married or the parent of a child 18 years old or younger. Those whose work problems interfered with family life were 3 times more likely to have a mood disorder, such as depression; 2.5 times more likely to have an

anxiety disorder; and 2 times more likely to have a substance
dependence disorder than those without conflicts.[27]

The amazing news from this study came when the researchers
examined the flip side of this issue. That is, what happens when
family problems interfered with work? Respondents who indicated this sort of stress were *30 times* more likely to have a mood
disorder, *9.5 times* more likely to have anxiety disorders, and
11 times more likely to have a substance dependence disorder
than those without family-to-work conflicts!

While it is clear that we should not overlook the impact that
work has on family, let us also remember to support each other's
work. Remember: A successful life is about love *and* work.

PARENTS AS PARTNERS, AND WITH AWARENESS

We have had the pleasure of working with many physicians who
reported high levels of satisfaction in both their marriage and
their relationships with their children. Many others, though, have
expressed the sentiment described by Jonah, a busy surgeon:

> "I feel like I'm 'on the sidelines' in my own family; I'm left out of the fiber and flow
> of family connection, because I'm so often away at work. And when I am around,
> my wife makes me feel like I don't know what I'm doing. She is clearly 'the family
> expert.' She knows everything imaginable about my kids. I don't. It's tough to feel
> motivated to make more time for family, when being with my family does not feel
> good to me."

The medical literature is amazingly devoid of helpful information
regarding how busy medical families deal with the joys and challenges of parenthood. In a forthcoming book, we will help to fill
this void. In conjunction with the American Medical Association
Alliance, we have conducted the largest-ever survey of physician
spouses, asking for input about a variety of "in-the-trenches"
issues, including parenting. We were still gathering data when
The Resilient Physician went to press, so no definitive analysis
from this project can yet be reported. However, an informal summary of key points made by the more than 400 surveys we have
received to date and observations from our family counseling
experiences with physician families are worth noting.

Share Responsibility; Don't Just "Help Out"

We intend for you to hear this bit of advice on several levels. First, accept that parenting is a joint responsibility. Even in a traditional marriage, when a father is conceptualized as "helping out" when he "baby-sits" or otherwise engages in some parenting role, it tends to perpetuate the notion that to be a father is to be a second-string parent.

We are not implying that resilient medical families accomplish the mythical 50/50 split in sharing parenting responsibilities. In truth, even in dual-career couples, one parent virtually always assumes the lion's share of responsibility for running home and hearth, and that person most often is the mother. However, it is also true that, when a dual-career couple becomes parents, resilience hinges on both partners making career sacrifices in order to orchestrate a greater level of sharing in domestic responsibilities than do traditional couples. Recent research by Sobecks et al[24] demonstrated that, when physicians marry each other, *both* spouses make career sacrifices in deference to family needs, even though "in dual-physician marriages, the professional family lives of both male and female physicians continue to reflect dominant gender roles."[24]

Second, for both mothers and fathers, it is important to accept responsibility for your relationship with your children, independent of your partner's level of involvement in hands-on parenting. Men: Don't fall prey to the notion that "parenting is mom's role." Women: Don't fall prey to the notion that "because dad is once again not here, we are an incomplete family."

In contrast to this latter sentiment, wives in resilient, traditional medical families tend to take the perspective suggested by one of the respondents to our AMA-Alliance Medical Marriage Survey:

> "I learned to accept that, much of the time, I would have to function independently from my husband. Often, I essentially feel like a single parent. But it has been important for me to accept, rather than to resent, this. When my husband is present, he can only be lovingly a part of our family if I am not harboring bitterness toward him in my heart."

Finally, it is essential that you share responsibility for keeping each other abreast of the details of your children's lives. Children feel closest to parents who know the details of their lives: what they feel, fear, enjoy, want, and need. Resilient medical parents make it a priority to solicit such information from their children and to share this information freely with each other.

Honor Each Other

Resilient medical families accept and honor each other's roles. Medical marriages with children who report high levels of happiness are amazingly lacking in rancor about their busy lives or about whatever role division they have implemented. In a healthy medical family, each parent's role is honored and respected by *both* partners. The spouse who does the bulk of the parenting does so with pride and acceptance of the important role he or she is playing, even at the price of having made career sacrifices. And the parent who is less involved is verbal about his or her appreciation and respect for the partner's contributions.

Similarly, rather than the classic mantra, "Your Dad is never here," the at-home spouse in a resilient medical marriage is careful to honor the relatively absent parent. This is done openly and consistently. Examples include complimenting and expressing support for and admiration for all that the busy physician-mate does.

A beautiful example of honoring came from a recent *JAMA* editorial, written by a nurse-daughter about her deceased physician-father:

"Other children's fathers played ball with them, took them camping and on vacations. . . . Paradoxically, it was my father's absences that taught me something more, a stratum above; the meaning of responsibility, a commitment to purpose, and the necessity in the adult world to reconcile oneself with grace early on to the inevitable tragic injustices of life."[28]

Give Up the Quest To Raise the Perfect Child

Every parent wants their children to grow up to become responsible adults. To this end, we educate them in the best schools possible. We teach them manners. We correct their grammar. We structure their activities. And on, and on, and on.

Let us not forget that one of the most powerful ways to help a child to develop a positive sense of self is to bless the child with the nurturing presence of parents. In our well-intended efforts to educate and enrich them, we sometimes contaminate our children's experiences with us. Regularly take a break from teaching your children. Let them see your human, playful side. In this regard, remember our aforementioned advice. If you spend long periods of time working, your child's collective memories of you will be skewed by his or her experiences on vacations or other times away from work. Do not make the mistake of contaminating these times with activities that stir your competitive, Type A coping habits. Rather, structure vacations and days off with your children doing things that allow you to relax and be enjoyable company for them.

Accept That Your Behavior Does Affect Your Children

When was the last time your morning family conversations sounded like this Dad or Mom: "I am so excited! I am looking forward to my day. I have a lot of great stuff waiting for me today. I've got a busy schedule filled with stuff that I love to do!"

Too often parents live in ways that convey to their children the message "This is what being a grown-up is like, kid: You get to choose between being stressed, anxious, guilty, angry, frazzled, fatigued, irritable, and fed up. Now, if you study hard, you will get to grow up and become like me."

Our advice to *both* parents: Avoid the "Pleasing Others, Even if It Kills Me or Them" syndrome.[1,10] Remember to check your Type A coping habits at the door when you arrive home in the evenings. You know that you are creating the wrong environment for your children if you find yourself doing any of the following:[10]

- Reacting to your child's behavior more often with criticism than with nurturing and praising
- Perceiving your children as stressors rather than as blessings
- Expressing approval to your child contingent on the child's performing in an exceptional manner in realms you deem important
- Attending only to the outcomes and not the process of your child's efforts
- Driving your children with life-scripting messages to "hurry up," "be perfect," and "get more aggressive"
- Generally modeling a Type A style of living

In this later regard, we have cautioned that children learn from how they are treated and what they observe.[10] Consider:

If the parent: lives in constant readiness, always alert for hidden challenges when dealing with others, struggles against time and other people, sets excessively rejoicing only when achievements are recognized by others and reproaches him or herself when they fail to meet perfectionistic standards

Then the child learns to: be hypervigilant and normalize such behavior, believe that life is a struggle, be driven and perfectionistic.

A few sobering questions can help keep you on track:

- Would your children and your family be better off with fewer activities and less "stuff" and calmer parents?
- Do you teach your children to fear "wasting time" and enjoying life?
- Do you maintain contact with your children by keeping up with who they know, what they do, what they like, and what they worry about?
- Are you creating family rituals that teach children to protect time for loved ones, even in a busy life?
- Are you teaching your children to be loyal to loved ones?
- Are you honest about the effects that your life is having on your children?
- Are you doing your fair share of the "in-the-trenches" parenting work?

Be Realistic

Having kids will diminish marital satisfaction, at least for a while. In the Olson and Olson[11] survey, 84% reported that having child(ren) reduced their marital satisfaction.

But recent data showed that having a strong foundation of friendship between spouses could increase marital satisfaction once a child arrives on the scene. Specifically, these researchers studied 82 couples for the first 4 to 6 years of their marriages. During that time, 43 couples became parents and 39 remained childless. Essentially, the researchers found that, although it is true that becoming parents stresses all couples, "happy marriages make for happy parents."[29]

Accept That Special Challenges Come When a Parent Is Gay or Lesbian

A homosexual parent who ends his or her heterosexual marriage and then reveals his or her homosexuality faces particular challenges. Such families tend to encounter exaggerated strains that are typical of stepfamilies. Ambiguity about parental roles and authority may prove to be confusing. The children may experience conflicts of loyalties that are exaggerated if anyone in the system shows intolerance or lack of acceptance of homosexuality.

If the gay or lesbian parent joins with a new partner, this "step" partner is likely to struggle to gain acceptance, both by the children and the ex-spouse and extended family. And the gay or lesbian partner may have difficulty coming to terms with the need to share his or her partner with others (ie, the partner's children). These stressors may take a serious toll on all involved as they try to establish a new norm for the stepfamily system.

Some estranged heterosexual ex-spouses express fear over having their children exposed to the "gay lifestyle." This despite the fact that impressive data from well-conducted research studies have documented that children reared by lesbian mothers and their partners are at no greater risk for psychiatric illness or gender identity and sexual-orientation problems than those raised by heterosexual couples.[30,31]

FIGHT TO KEEP YOUR RELATIONSHIP ALIVE

Few factors promote stress resilience more than a loving, intimate lifetime partnership. We believe passionately that such relationships are worth fighting for. To do so requires that you regularly create contexts that give three things a chance to grow: your friendship, your communication, and your romance. Many of the tools and strategies that we have already outlined can help. We add here encouragement to regularly and directly discuss your problems.

Avoidance—failure to openly address your conflicts—is one of the key relationship patterns that is predictive of unhappiness and divorce.[32] Prospective studies[33] of married couples have shown that all married couples—those who are happily married and those who end their marriage in divorce—frequently squabble. But two factors distinguish happy couples from those who divorce or otherwise live in misery: (1) how the partners behave when they have conflict and (2) how they behave when they are not in conflict. Let us elaborate.

What to Avoid

Don't let your communication kill your friendship and intimacy. The preeminent marital researcher, psychologist John Gottman of the University of Washington, demonstrated in his prospective studies that couples who eventually divorce tend to accumulate tensions due to predictable, avoidable patterns of interaction that become habitual. According to Gottman, the following behaviors are to be avoided when dealing with conflict:[33]

- *Waiting too long before bringing up what is bothering you.* Doing so results in the proverbial "hot start-up" wherein the opening salvo is a critical attack on one's partner. Interestingly, according to Gottman, women tend to engage in hot start-ups far more frequently than do men, probably because they are prone to tolerate frustrations, hoping they will dwindle. Instead, the frustrations fester into resentments, resulting in explosions like, "You are never here! I'm sick and tired of this!" Far better to regularly express what's bothering you, minus some of the volume and rancor.

- *Reacting to your partner's concerns with defensiveness.* Even a hot start-up is fueled by pain. Learn to respond to your partner's underlying issue and to separate the person from the problem being addressed. Details on how to negotiate conflict without damaging your relationship are presented in Chapter 8.

- *Showing contempt.* Productive communication is killed and the soul of your marriage is damaged if you act as though you feel contempt for your partner. Dysfunctional couples convey contempt when they argue by using sarcasm, cynicism, mockery, hostile humor, or other forms of conveying disgust.

- *Stonewalling.* Contempt and defensiveness tend to perpetuate each other. Couples who communicate in these ways get stuck in self-perpetuating, downward spirals of interaction. Often, the next step in this deadly dance is stonewalling, which is a form of disengaging from conflict by avoiding not only this discussion but the marriage itself. According to Gottman's research, this behavior is far more common in men.

■ *Failed repair attempts.* A repair attempt is "any statement or action. . .that prevents negativity from escalating out of control."[33] These are the efforts that couples make to de-escalate tension during arguments, to take a break and calm down. If repair attempts drop out of a couple's way of interacting or if one partner decides to no longer respond to the other's efforts at repair, contempt and defensiveness rein. The result is that the partners feel "flooded" with each other's negativity. This is not only a state of emotional discomfort; as we discuss following, this can also be dangerous to your health.

Jan Kiecolt-Glaser and Ron Glaser of Ohio State are a husband-and-wife research team who have studied the physiological consequences of marital interactions. In a recent study of 97 happily married newlyweds, the researchers found that when couples engaged in high levels of abrasive behaviors, they suffered serious physiological consequences.[34] Specifically, Kiecolt-Glaser and colleagues found that, for both husbands and wives, behaviors like criticizing, disagreeing, denying responsibility, making excuses, interrupting, making put-downs, and trying to coerce the other into concurring lead to significant spikes in blood pressure and heart rate and plummeted measures of immune system functions to levels far lower than those measured in couples who did not show such abrasive behaviors. A follow-up study with older couples married an average of 42 years found that females, especially, experienced many endocrine changes following a marital argument.[35]

Other researchers[33] report that during conflict or emotional stress, a man's blood pressure and heart rate rise much higher and stay elevated longer than his wife's does. And psychologist Tim Smith of the University of Utah noted that the higher the hostility level, the larger the blood pressure surge when married couples discuss a topic about which they disagree.[36]

If these communication mistakes become habitual, your relationship will fill with more negative than positive sentiment. Soon, for both emotional and physiological reasons, partners in such a conflict-laden relationship become triggers of alarm for each other, rather than generating feelings associated with well-being. The stage is then set for explosive interactions, even in response to relatively benign and commonplace irritants that otherwise would go unnoticed as you move through your busy life.

Special Challenges of Gay and Lesbian Medical Couples

For some gay or lesbian couples, drama around "coming out" strains the relationship from its outset. Coming out refers to the process of accepting a homosexual identity. It begins with self-acceptance then includes disclosure to others of one's choosing. Gay males and lesbians vary tremendously along the axis of self-acceptance and comfort with self-disclosure, and differences between couple members on either of these dimensions can prove to be quite stressful to the relationship.

Once established, gay and lesbian couples may face further challenges that distinguish them from other medical couples. For many, dealing with social prejudice and lack of support for relationship issues is a primary stressor. For example, in a survey of women physicians (aged 30–70 years) from the Women Physicians Health Study, lesbians were 4 times more likely than heterosexual physicians to report ever having experienced sexual orientation-based harassment in a medical setting.[37] And a recent survey of 500 people living in an urban Canadian city found that nearly 12% stated that they would refuse to see a gay or lesbian family physician.[38]

This latter statistic may seem negligible to someone who has never suffered discrimination. But clinical experiences with gay, lesbian, and bisexual physicians and their loved ones has underscored that any act of discrimination or lack of support or acceptance of their lifestyle is hurtful and can compound already high levels of stress for these couples and families. In this regard, Burke et al[39] reminded us that gay, lesbian, and bisexual physicians face painful obstacles similar to any other minority group within the profession. Lack of acceptance from community, families, and acquaintances at work can result in loneliness and a sense of isolation.

Most gay male and lesbian couples do not have children as a common central focus. Therefore, they do not have a built-in, pervasive shared purpose, "a generative extension of themselves."[40] In some cases, the absence of children or supportive extended family leaves a gay or lesbian couple feeling that they must be "all things to each other," a dynamic that can prove to be smothering of individuality.

On the positive side, psychiatrist Michael Myers[40] pointed out that, compared to heterosexual relationships, gay and lesbian relationships are more commonly structured along egalitarian lines. Both partners are afforded equal power. In traditional marriages, on the other hand, there is more often a power differential; the primary breadwinner holds more power.

Clinical anecdotal experience has suggested that, with gay male couples, competition with each other is a common complaint and a destructive relationship element. According to Myers,[40] competition is both the cause and result of other problems in the relationship. Competitiveness can lead to feeling unsupported and distanced from one's partner. Unfortunately, this same lack of support is likely to bring out a competitive need to bolster one's self-pride and self-esteem through competition about money, intelligence, success in the job market, sports, looks, or sexual prowess.

According to Roth,[41] the universal relationship dilemma of how one can find a middle ground that comfortably balances togetherness and individual autonomy can be especially difficult for many lesbian couples. Clinical experience suggests that this is a less prominent problem in lesbian couples who are blessed with accepting communities and extended families and who are integrated in the lesbian and heterosexual communities.

Follow the "Intimacy Formula"

If you want to keep friendship and intimacy alive, you have to do more than simply avoid problem styles of communicating. A distinguishing feature of happy couples is how they treat each other when they are not having conflict.[1,10,11,32,33] Specifically, resilient couples make it a habit to regularly interact in ways that are positive. Put another way, they make it a habit to catch each other doing things right, to compliment each other, to express appreciation, and to otherwise honor each other—even during those stretches of time when they are intermittently struggling with some issue. In fact, based on their analysis of a longitudinal study of more than 2,000 married couples, Gottman and Silver[42] claimed that happy couples on average have 5 times as many positive interactions and expressions as negative interactions and expressions.

We close this section with 11 recommendations for keeping intimacy alive.[1,10] Each strategy can be considered a single "ingredient" in a formula for intimacy. Do these habitually, and you are likely to keep your communication, your friendship, and your romance alive.

1. *Protect your communication-generating rituals.* Every couple starts out with a wonderful set of rituals that create time and space for them to give undivided attention to each other. What were yours? Healthy medical couples don't do anything extraordinary here. After all, no one wants to spend hours each day discussing his or her innermost insecurities and fears. (Most of us would rather have a root canal!)

   The "rituals" that thriving couples maintain are much smaller, much more gentle and realistic. Maybe it's taking time to leisurely read the Sunday paper—not in parallel silence, but together, interacting about interesting points. Some develop the habit of setting aside 20 minutes each evening to sit and chat in a quiet room. Others make mealtime a time to sit at the table for an extra 15 minutes, just to touch base. Still others protect their weekly walks together, their Tuesday night "recesses" (no working, no worrying, no discussing anything "heavy"). It doesn't matter *how* you do it, *just do it!*

2. *Practice the basics of effective communication.* At the risk of redundancy, we reiterate this important point: If you want to keep intimacy alive, it is not enough just to "show up"; you have to behave (ie, communicate) in ways that connect you with your partner. Remember these seven essentials to good communication:[43]

   - Learn to listen
   - Be aware of the nonverbal message
   - Learn to communicate your feelings
   - Use "I" statements; avoid accusatory "you" statements and "why" questions
   - Learn to be a compassionate, reflective listener
   - Agree not to attack the other person or to defend yourself when your partner is expressing a concern
   - Have regular couple-communication times

3. *Continue to get to know each other.* Every week, learn something new about your partner. "If you are not learning something new about each other, you are not paying close enough attention."[1]

4. *Take a night off approximately each week to meander with each other.* As hard as you both work, you certainly can afford to take a little recess. On these evenings, resist the temptation to engage in those subtle forms of work that keep you from relaxing: checking e-mail or voice mail at work, doing that extra load of laundry, reading work-related material. Remember: Taking "recess" is supposed to be about having fun. Practice doing so until you get good at it.

5. *Each month, protect a 12- to 48-hour period of time to escape together.* Use this time to renew your nurturing, affectionate attention to each other.

6. *Regularly give each other personal surprises.* In constructing these, be sure to consider *your partner's needs and likes.* For example, even if you are comfortable getting away for a weekend, if your partner is anxious about work-related or childcare responsibilities, the wonderful surprise of "kidnapping" them for a romantic getaway will only work if you have done the footwork required to make sure their anxieties are soothed.

7. *Remember to be open, playful, and flexible in your sexual relationship.* Be realistic here: The stresses and demands of your life (and aging) may change your sexual patterns. But remember that research with couples under the age of 60 has shown that frequency of sexual relations does not correlate with subjectively determined levels of satisfaction with one's sex life. Rather, the couple's level of comfort discussing their sexual relationship with each other is the crucial determiner of their satisfaction.[44] In addition, a couple's level of mutual satisfaction with the amount of affection they show each other has been shown to be one of the most powerful discriminators between happily and unhappily married couples. Specifically, in 72% of happily married couples, partners reported being satisfied with the physical affection they get from each other, versus only 28% of unhappy couples.[11]

8. *Reaffirm your permission and encouragement to grow as individuals.* "Romance blossoms in relationships that free the individuals

to be fully expressive of their respective selves."[1] For most couples, this means repeatedly adjusting to new "steps" thrown into their relationship dances as first one then the other of you changes in the infinite ways compelled by human development. Resist any temptation to think (or to scream) "double-crossed!" or "midlife crisis!" at such times. Rather, react with inquisitiveness. Find out what this new aspect of your partner is all about.

Once the kids are grown, medical couples face new opportunities and challenges. The second half of marriage is a time to look back with pride on what you have done and what you have endured; to forgive each other for mistakes you've made; to find new ways to spend time together; to disinhibit your sexual relationship; to renew your friendship; to establish new levels of nurturing companionship with your grown children; and to notice and express appreciation anew for all that your partner does and has done for you and your family.[43] Of course, younger medical couples are well-advised not to wait until retirement to enjoy the many intimacy-boosters we are discussing.

9. *Apologize and forgive.* There are no perfect people. There are no perfect marriages or families. Along the journey that is a lifetime marriage, we make many mistakes, we encounter many disappointments, and we regularly fail to please those we most love. This is just as true for thriving medical couples as it is for those who divorce. But resilient medical couples make it a habit to regularly apologize and forgive.

10. *Believe together.* Contemporary researchers have shown similarity in spiritual beliefs is a characteristic of resilient couples. In Chapter 4 we discussed the fact that belief in God is a resilience-booster for individuals. Here, we emphasize that families that pray and worship together and couples that come from similar religious traditions are more likely to remain united and to report higher levels of happiness than those without such beliefs or shared traditions.[45]

11. *Hang in there!* Remember: It's never too early or too late to make your marriage better.

In *The Case for Marriage,* University of Chicago professor Linda Waite and Director of the Marriage Program at the Institute of American Values Maggie Gallagher tout the many advantages that a good marriage brings, including enhanced health, productivity, and happiness.[46] Further, they cite research that shows that, just as good marriages go bad, bad marriages "go good." Five years after reporting high levels of marital unhappiness, 86% of continuously married couples that stayed married now called their marriage either "very happy" or "quite happy."

BE GENEROUS AND BE GRACIOUS

We most often close our lectures on medical marriage by reminding audiences that virtually all advice about how to make marriage work can be subsumed under two factors: Loving medical families treat each other with generosity and graciousness.

Be generous in what you offer to your loved ones. Offer them "gifts" that make them feel safe and special in your presence, even if offering their preferred forms of communication, affection, or attention feels awkward for you. And *be gracious* when responding to the "gifts" your loved ones offer to you, even if the offering is not exactly what you wished for.

CONCLUSIONS

The work–family challenges faced by physicians are unique and extraordinary. Unfortunately, support for managing these challenges is too often lacking, both in our culture at large and within the medical subculture.

This is unfortunate, given that the benefits of even brief, psychoeducationally oriented relationship counseling have been indisputably demonstrated. For example, a 5-year prospective, controlled study[47] demonstrated the efficacy of a five-session training in communication and conflict management.

Our consulting experiences attest to the fact that physicians respond positively when psychoeducational programs are incorporated into their typical continuing education curricula. In addition, excellent self-help resources that teach positive skills for enhancing marriage and family life are available.[1,10,11,32,33,48]

If we are to stay the course and remain stress resilient at work and at home, we must find ways to keep our marriage and family relationships healthy; doing so is the ultimate act of heroism.

REFERENCES—CHAPTER 5

1. Sotile WM, Sotile MO. *The Medical Marriage: Sustaining Healthy Relationships for Physicians and Their Families.* Chicago, Ill: American Medical Association; 2000.

2. Crane M. Getting personal: Who is today's doctor, anyway? *Med Econ.* November 2000:2–3.

3. Peterson KS. 2001 people to watch. *USA Today.* December 27, 2000; 8D.

4. Walsh F. The concept of family resilience: Crisis and challenge. *Family Process.* 1996;35:261–281.

5. Werner EE. Risk, resilience, and recovery: Perspectives from the Kauai Longitudinal Study. *Dev Psychopathol.* 1993;5:503–515.

6. Coyne J, DeLongis A. Going beyond social support: The role of social relationships in adaptation. *J Consult Clin Psychol.* 1986;54:454–460.

7. Ornstein R, Sobel D. *Healthy Pleasures.* Reading, Mass: Addison-Wesley; 1989.

8. Chambers R, Campbell I. Anxiety and depression in general practitioners: Associations with type of practice, fundholding, gender and other personal characteristics. *Family Practice.* 1996;13: 170–173.

9. Williams R, Williams V. *Life-Skills.* New York, NY: Time Books; 1997.

10. Sotile WM, Sotile MO. *Beat Stress Together.* New York, NY: John Wiley & Sons; 1999.

11. Olson DH, Olson AK. *Empowering Couples: Building on Your Strengths,* 2nd ed. Minneapolis, Minn: Life Innovations, Inc; 2000.

12. Csikszentmihalyi M. *Finding Flow.* New York, NY: Basic Books; 1997.

13. Frankel P. Time and couples, part II: The sixty-second pleasure point. In: Nelson TS, Trepper TS, eds. *101 More Interventions in Family Therapy.* New York, NY: The Haworth Press; 1998:145–149.

14. Babitsky S, Mangraviti JJ. *The Successful Physician Negotiator: How to Get What You Deserve.* Falmouth, Mass: SEAK, Inc; 1998.

15. Waters D, Saunders JT. I gave at the office. *Family Therapy Networker;* 1996;20(2):44–51.

16. Brunicardi FC, Hobson FL. Time management: A review for physicians. *J Natl Med Assoc.* 1996;88:561–587.

17. *Medical Economics.* November 2000;19: entire issue.

18. Jackson SE, Maslach C. After-effects of job-related stress: Families as victims. *J Occup Behav.* 1982;3:63–77.

19. Larson R, Richards MH. *Divergent Realities: The Emotional Lives of Mothers, Fathers, and Adolescents.* New York, NY: Basic Books; 1994.

20. Ducker D. Research on women physicians with multiple roles: A feminist perspective. *JAMWA*. 1994;49:78–84.

21. Levinson W, Kaufman K, Tolle SW. Women in academic medicine: Strategies for balancing career and personal life. *JAMWA*. 1992;47:25–29.

22. Carnes M. Balancing family and career: Advice from the trenches. *Ann Intern Med*. 1996;125:618–620.

23. Law JK. Starting a family in medical school. *JAMA*. 1997;277:767.

24. Sobecks NW, Justice AC, Hinze S, et al. When doctors marry doctors: A survey exploring the professional and family lives of young physicians. *Ann Intern Med*. 1999;130:312–319.

25. Thornton J. *Chore Wars: How Households Can Share the Work and Keep the Peace*. Berkeley, Calif: Conari Press; 1993.

26. Landau C, Hall S, Wartman SA, Macko MB. Stress in social and family relationships during the medical residency. *J Med Educ*. 1986;61:654–660.

27. Frone MR. Work–family conflict and employee psychiatric disorders: The National Comorbidity Survey. *J Appl Psychol*. 2000;85:888–895.

28. Hermann E. A piece of my mind: Father's day. *JAMA*. 1990;263:3017.

29. Shapiro AF, Gottman JM, Carrere S. The baby and the marriage: Identifying factors that buffer against decline in marital satisfaction after the first baby arrives. *J Fam Psychol*. 2000;14:59-70.

30. Golombok S, Spenser A, Rutter M. Children in lesbian and single-parent households: Psychosexual and psychiatric appraisal. *J Child Psychol Psychiatry*. 1983;24:551–572.

31. Green R. The best interests of the child with a lesbian mother. *Bull AAPL*. 1982;10:7–15.

32. Markman H, Stanley S, Blumberg SL. *Fighting for Your Marriage*. San Francisco, Calif: Jossey-Bass; 1994.

33. Gottman JM, Silver N. *The Seven Principles for Making Marriage Work*. New York, NY: Three Rivers Press; 1999.

34. Kiecolt-Glaser JK, Malarkey W, Chee MA, Newton T, Cacioppo JT, Mao HY, Glaser R. Negative behavior during marital conflict is associated with immunological down-regulation. *Psychosom Med*. 1993;55:395–409.

35. Kiecolt-Glaser JK, Glaser R, Cacioppo JT, MacCallum RC, Syndersmith M, Kim C, Malarkey WB. Marital conflict in older adults: Endocrinological and immunological correlates. *Psychosom Med*. 1997;59:339–349.

36. Smith TW, Allred KD. Blood pressure reactivity during social interaction in high and low cynical hostile men. *J Behav Med.* 1989;11:135–143.

37. Brogan DJ, Frank E, Elon L, Sivanesan P, O'Hanlan KA. Harassment of lesbians as medical students and physicians. *JAMA.* 1999;282:1290–1292.

38. Druzin P, Shrier I, Yacowar M, Rossignol M. Discrimination against gay, lesbian and bisexual family physicians by patients. *Can Med Assoc J.* 1998;158:593–597.

39. Burke BP, White JC. Well-being of gay, lesbian, and bisexual doctors. *BMJ.* 2001;322:422.

40. Myers MF. *Doctors' Marriages: A Look at the Problems and Their Solutions.* New York, NY: Plenum; 1988.

41. Roth S. Psychotherapy with lesbian couples: Individual issues, female socialization, and the social context. *J Marital Fam Ther.* 1985;11:273–286.

42. Gottman JM, Silver N. *Why Marriages Succeed or Fail: What You Can Learn from the Breakthrough Research to Make Your Marriage Last.* New York, NY: Simon and Schuster; 1994.

43. Arp D, Arp C. *The Second Half of Marriage.* Grand Rapids, Mich: Zondervan Publishing House; 1996.

44. Laumann EO, Michael RT, Gagnon JH, Michaels S. *The Social Organization of Sexuality: Sexual Practices in the United States.* Chicago, Ill: University of Chicago Press; 1994.

45. Mahoney A, Pargament TJ, Swank AB, Scott E, Emery E, Rye M. Marriage and the spiritual realm: The role of proximal and distal religious constructs in marital functioning. *J Fam Psychol.* 1999;13:321–338.

46. Waite LJ, Gallagher M. *The Case for Marriage: Why Married People are Happier, Healthier, and Better Off Financially.* New York, NY: Doubleday; 2000.

47. Markman HJ, Renick MJ, Floyd FJ, Stanley SM, Clements M. Preventing marital distress through communication and conflict management training: A 4- and 5-year follow-up. *J Consult Clin Psychol.* 1993;61:70–77.

48. Hendrix H. *Getting the Love You Want: A Guide for Couples.* New York, NY: Harper & Row; 1990.

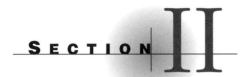

SECTION II

Understanding and Managing Relationships in the Medical Workplace

Conflict Self-Assessment

"In the day-to-day world, no intelligence is more important than the interpersonal."

Daniel Goleman
Emotional Intelligence[1] (p. 42)

L et's begin with a fantasy exercise. Pretend that it is our mission to create a context that is sure to breed interpersonal conflict. If we combine the following ingredients, we are sure to accomplish our goal:

1. Involve a number of high-powered, opinionated, turf-protecting parties.
2. Create uncertainty about options and outcomes in areas that matter to the parties involved.
3. Make sure that the exact nature of the organization's processes and the personal agendas of the various players remain vague.
4. Make competition and evaluation an integral part of your interpersonal culture.
5. Add heaping doses of stress and pressure.
6. Threaten or actually impart negative consequences to all parties involved.
7. Put all of the above in a context of change.

This scenario may at first sound unlikely. But if you examine it closely, you will probably find it to be alarmingly familiar. Whether at work or home, most physicians live with this formula for conflict. Is it any wonder that many physicians today have difficulty maintaining harmonious relationships?

No discussion of emotional well-being for physicians can be complete without examining interpersonal conflict. Proficiency in conflict management and dispute resolution is an essential part of the modern physician's coping toolbox. Unfortunately, the coping strategies that make for a successful physician may work against your ability to effectively resolve conflict. Leonard Marcus, Director of the Program for Health Care Negotiation and Conflict Resolution at the Harvard School of Public Health, noted that many physicians, especially those in positions of authority, " believe the best way to resolve conflict is through adversarial methods."[2 (p. 9)] Adds his colleague, physician and conflict management consultant Barry Dorn, "As physicians, we're very used to being prescriptive—we're presented information and we say, 'Okay, here's the answer to the problem.'"[2 (p. 11)] Unfortunately, when dealing with collegial tensions, physicians may disagree about what is the right "prescription" to remedy their differences. At this point, the ability to negotiate a resolution of the conflict becomes a necessary skill if goodwill in the relationship is to be maintained.

In this chapter, we help you examine your personal conflict management style and discuss what may be hindering your ability to effectively negotiate conflict. We present tools that can help you assess the stages of conflict in your organization or relationship and your own conflict style. We also offer tips for conflict prophylaxis.

WHO ARE YOU TO OTHERS?

Interpersonal dynamics involve at least three dimensions: What I show to other people (ie, my interpersonal "posture"); the role I see myself playing in the relationship; and my private feelings about the relationship.[3] Use the three scales in Exercises 6-1 and 6-2 to get a broad-stroke assessment of both your professional and personal relationships.

The crucial question is what are you doing to move your relationships toward the right side of each of these scales? If you're like many physicians, the answer is "not much." We often see a paradox in high-performing people. On the one hand, they behave in take-charge ways that are quite impressive. But when conflict hits, they assume an atypically passive, passive–aggressive, or otherwise ineffectual stance. Soon, the actual relationship, and not the problems that caused the relationship conflict, becomes the problem.

EXERCISE 6-1

Scale Regarding Your Professional Relationships

Instructions: On the following scales, check the words that best describe your PROFESSIONAL relationships.

My Interpersonal Posture

At work, I tend to "show" other people . . .

rage—resentment—anger—frustration—MIDPOINT—engagement—enthusiasm—free-flowing interchange—shared passion for a mutual goal—friendliness—affection

How I View My Role

Regarding my role within my organization, I see myself as being . . .

martyred—lacking trust of others—jealous of others—envious of others—blaming of others—feeling sorry for myself —being misunderstood—MIDPOINT—curious—open to input—accepting my fair share of responsibility—having faith in others—trusting of others—a source of creative collaboration

My Private Emotions

Overall, what I generally feel when I'm at work is . . .

rage—panic—dread—anxiety—fear—frustration—MIDPOINT—concern—empathy—compassion—respect—enthusiasm—optimism—joy

We believe that this insidious process threatens the stress resilience of many physicians. In today's medical marketplace, conflict seems to be inevitable. It comes in many flavors: conflict between physicians and nurses, conflict between physicians and medical or insurance company administrators, and/or conflict between physicians and their physician colleagues.

We do not mean to imply that all physicians are miserable. To the contrary, many physicians we know enjoy extraordinarily collegial relationships. Although no empirical validation of our belief on this matter exists, we suspect that the approximately 65% of the physician population sampled who report high levels of career satisfaction[4,5] are, for the most part, those physicians who manage their relationships in positive ways. Our concern is for those who do not. Again, our hypothesis awaits empirical verification, but this observation is unquestionably reliable across our

---

E x e r c i s e 6-2

Scale Regarding Your Most Important Personal Relationships

Instructions: On the following scales, check the words that best describe your most important PERSONAL relationship. (Note: You may want to repeat this exercise for several different relationships.)

My Interpersonal Posture

When I am with _____ (name the person), I tend to "show" . . .

rage—resentment—anger—frustration—MIDPOINT—engagement—enthusiasm—free-flowing interchange—shared passion for a mutual goal—friendliness—affection—love

How I View My Role

Regarding my role within my relationship with _____ (name the person), I see myself as being. . .

martyred—lacking trust—jealous—envious—blaming—feeling sorry for myself—being misunderstood—MIDPOINT—curious—open to input—accepting my fair share of responsibility—having faith in the relationship—-trusting this person—a source of creative collaboration

My Private Emotions

Overall, what I generally feel when I am with _____ (name the person) is. . .

rage—panic—dread—anxiety—fear—frustration—MIDPOINT—concern—empathy—compassion—respect—enthusiasm—optimism—joy—love

---

clinical experiences: We have never met a physician dissatisfied with his or her career who did not complain of strained relationships with colleagues.

If managed appropriately, conflict is an opportunity for growth, a way of forging new understandings and greater levels of trust and respect for each other. But mismanaged conflict functions like a festering abscess in a relationship; its toxic effects eventually damage health, morale, and productivity for all parties concerned.

WHAT IS YOUR CONFLICT MANAGEMENT STYLE?

Kilmann and Thomas'[6] seminal conceptualization of five conflict management styles remains one of the most helpful heuristics available in this field of study. Aschenbrener and Siders[3] and Waitley[7] offered concise summaries of the pros and cons of each of the five strategies outlined by Kilmann and Thomas. As you read through the following descriptions, note your own management style. It might also prove helpful to note the styles of other people—those you get along with comfortably and those with whom you tend to struggle.

Dominator

Here, individuals compete to overcome and dominate the opposition. Behavior is fueled by the underlying assumption that conflict is a contest in which one either wins or loses.

Pros: Dominator strategies may be necessary and appropriate when:

- Resources in question cannot be divided (eg, when pursuing a true win/lose endeavor, like a research grant that will be awarded to only one applicant)
- The issue is compliance with a high-stakes policy (eg, sexual harassment)
- Significant time constraints limit the process (eg, when managing life-or-death medical crises)
- The other party refuses to take anything other than a competitive approach

Cons: The competitive juices that dominators thrive on and stir in others do not make for collaborative relationships. Dominators typically have difficulty rallying support for implementation of their decisions or ideas, even when they are right. The dominator's win/lose approach and willingness to do whatever it takes to "win," may result in won wars but lost battles (ie, damaged relationships).

Avoider

Sometimes called withdrawers, avoiders remove themselves from conflict, especially when they perceive themselves to be at risk of losing. Here, we see many of the "hit-and-run" strategies that busy physicians often use.[8] Because they are uncomfortable dealing directly with others, avoiders tend to store up resentments and then periodically flare. A flurry of conflict is followed by withdrawal into busyness, silence, or passive–aggressive resistance to any effort by the other party to directly engage them in open conflict resolution.

> *Pros:* Avoiding engagement in conflict is appropriate when winning is impossible or when a temporary cool-down period is advisable. This is an effective way to at least temporarily delay unpleasant, direct dealings with others. Avoidance is also appropriate if the conflict is trivial; it may be akin to a "live-and-let-live" attitude.

> *Cons:* In a brewing conflict, the more you avoid, the more likely it is that you will lose and that tension and resentment will build in the relationship. Avoiders miss opportunities to clarify issues, and unaddressed issues may trigger additional conflict. If you repeatedly avoid, others may come to think of you as weak and may lose confidence and esteem for you.

Compromiser

Compromisers work to get both parties to make some trade-offs and to get some of what they want. This is a back-up strategy when collaboration fails.

> *Pros:* Compromising is the appropriate style when both the issues and the relationship of the parties are important or when an expedient resolution that does not undermine implementation is needed. "Compromise may be used to achieve a temporary settlement of complex issues that require collaboration for long-term management."[2 (p. 46)]

> *Cons:* If you habitually go for compromise, you may fail to clarify underlying issues and may miss solutions that are better than the position of any single party. Also, it is often difficult to negotiate a compromise that truly balances the concessions so that all parties feel they have won and lost equally. Finally,

chronically compromising may breed frustration. As conflict management expert Denis Waitly succinctly put it: "Compromisers are invested in resolving conflict by negotiating an outcome in which both people feel equally unhappy."[7 (p. 13)]

Accommodator

Lessening of conflict and making others happy are the primary goals of accommodators (sometimes called placators). To do so, accommodators routinely subordinate their personal interests for the sake of preserving the relationship.

Pros: Accommodation is especially appropriate when:
- The issue at hand is much more important to the other party and you value the relationship more than the issue. (Example: You might decide to withdraw your name from the ballot in a race for an office because it is clear that winning is more important to a colleague.)
- You are in error or feel you can't win a competition.

Cons: If you habitually accommodate, you become easy prey for unscrupulous negotiators who do not differentiate truly important from unimportant issues. Accommodators are vulnerable to feeling steamrolled by the self-serving agendas of others, especially when dealing with those who use dominator strategies.

Collaborator

Often termed win–win, this style focuses on achieving goals rather than meeting demands. Collaboration grows from and fosters an understanding of complex issues and interdependent systems.

Pros: Collaboration is by far the most powerful way to devise creative solutions to problems. It builds consensus that ensures that all involved parties will cooperate with the implementation of the solutions. Collaboration is the road to creating sustainable change.

Cons: Collaboration takes a great deal of effort. It is time-consuming and requires that all parties listen and work together. Collaboration requires that both parties participate in good faith and invest in negotiating positive outcomes to their conflict.

A Caveat

Our work with medical organizations has led us to conceptualize that, in its extreme, mismanaged conflict festers into a sixth pattern: the disruptor syndrome. As of the mid to late 1990s, the problems of "disruptive physicians" became a frequent topic in the popular medical management literature. We have proposed that these problems cannot be effectively addressed by blaming or pathologizing physicians. Rather, a systemic view that understands disruptive behavior in the context of the relationship dynamics in which the physician is embroiled is necessary.[9] We close this chapter with discussion of various systemic factors that might lead to conflict in the medical workplace, but we defer targeted discussion of the disruptive physician syndrome to Chapter 9.

WHAT ARE YOUR HURDLES TO BECOMING AN EFFECTIVE NEGOTIATOR?

Consultant Roger Dawson[10] contends that, regardless of your individual conflict management style, eight factors leave physicians, as a group, remarkably ill-equipped to become good negotiators. We review these factors here in hopes of helping you to identify your problem areas.

1. *Physicians may feel that most negotiating tactics are unethical.*
   Unprincipled negotiators use a strategy that gives all negotiators a bad name: They severely overstate their initial demands, intending to reach a fall-back "compromise" that really was their original goal. To a physician who is trained to be truthful, this smacks of shady dealings.
2. *Physicians have been trained not to reveal emotions.* There is certainly nothing wrong with remaining calm during negotiations. In fact, most of the time, doing so is advantageous. But showing upset can also be an effective and powerful negotiating technique, one that many physicians find to be disconcerting.
3. *Physicians are trained to deal in reality, not perceptions.*
   Dawson[10 (p. 43)] contends that "The most important thing that you can do in a negotiation is to service the perception in the other person's mind that you have options." For a busy, forthright physician, "servicing perceptions" may seem like a petty manipulation and a waste of time and energy.

4. *Physicians are trained to gather facts before determining solutions.* Although steadfastness is a worthwhile strategy when time allows, negotiating during relationship crisis requires a different strategy. During times of crisis, effective negotiators look for solutions first, rather than gathering all the relevant facts before taking action. They utilize the "ready, fire, aim" approach, then clean up the relationship consequences. This method of negotiation stirs discomfort in physicians who are careful, deliberate, or obsessive in their interpersonal dealings.

5. *Physicians are conflict adverse.* If we know anything about the psychology of physicians, we know that, as a group, physicians tend to be invested in pleasing others. They want to make things better. This same psychodynamic that makes for a nice person can compromise a physician's power to negotiate. Effective negotiation requires the capacity to tolerate the anxiety that comes with the other person's distress about not getting their way. Courtesy and professionalism are certainly assets during any negotiation, but the ability to tolerate disagreement is a necessary part of most, if not all, successful negotiations.[11]

6. *Physicians don't like to lose.* Effective negotiators often use the leverage of being willing to walk away from the table. To do so involves bearing through an ostensible "loss" by giving up the struggle. Many physicians are so averse to "losing" that they never view "quitting" as a healthy choice. This hard-headed willingness to keep trying at all costs can compromise one's negotiating effectiveness. A frequent variant of this hurdle comes in the form of difficulty apologizing or admitting mistakes. Defensive dealings with others who deserve an apology simply fuel further conflict.

7. *Physicians may feel that it's beneath them to do anything for money.* Never before in the history of medicine have physicians been so frequently called on to negotiate issues that involve money. Many feel that doing so reduces the nobility of their profession to the status of a business. Reticence of this sort creates vulnerability when dealing with business persons who are congruently focused on negotiating the best possible financial deal for their side of the bargain. This same reticence may keep a physician from openly negotiating an employment contract that is truly acceptable to him or her. When this

occurs, subsequent resentments can set the tone for unex-
plained, strained relationships within the group.

8. *Physicians generally do not feel credentialed to negotiate.* "Like a
babe in the woods." These words succinctly describe the feeling many physicians report when they attempt to negotiate
financial and business matters with administrators or business leaders. Even more frequently, physicians are left to
flounder through tense interchanges with disgruntled
patients, staff, or colleagues. Unfortunately, traditional
medical education devotes little if any attention to teaching
physicians how to negotiate outcomes that will affect their
personal quality of life.

HOW ARE *YOU* DOING?

In any ongoing relationship, disagreements are inevitable. Conflict,
on the other hand, is optional.

The Stages of Conflict Scale,[7,9] presented in Exercise 6-3, can
help you to do two things: First, assess the status of any relationship and, second, identify how disagreements can escalate into
conflict. As you read through the scale, note that if you can simply agree to disagree when you encounter differences of opinion,
needs, or interpretations of facts, you can negotiate without damaging your relationship (Stage I).

Trouble comes when a mentality of scarcity sets in (Stage II):
Fearing that there is not enough of some valued commodity to go
around (eg, referrals, fame, money, power, attention, prestige, or
the status of being "right"), competitive attitudes begin to fuel
suspicious and defensive behaviors. Soon the other person is seen
to be the problem. This change in perspective leads to defensiveness, withholding of positive regard, and competitiveness. When
a win–lose mentality sets in (Stage III), factions solidify and
attempts begin to hurt or eliminate the other party or certain
members of the organization. The relationship system then
becomes stuck in toxic conflict that threatens the viability of the
relationship or the group.

If your responses suggest that your relationship is drifting
toward Stage II, take stock and commit yourself to aborting any
behavior that might push you into Stage III conflict. Tips on how
to do this will follow shortly.

E X E R C I S E   6-3

The Stages of Conflict Scale

Check items that apply to your organization or family. Total the checks at each stage of conflict.

Stage I: Agreeing to Disagree

__ Willing to meet and discuss facts

__ A cooperative spirit prevails

__ Issues can be discussed without involving personalities

__ The language used is specific

__ There is a sense of optimism

__ There is a "live-and-let-live" attitude

__ Parties are able to stay in the present tense

__ Solutions dominate your management efforts

__ *Total Stage I Characteristics*

Stage II: Conflict Begins to Heat Up the System

__ A competitive attitude predominates

__ Talk about problems, target people as being the problem

__ Frequent use of statements like "They," "You always, and and "He never" are heard

__ A "cover-your-rear" attitude predominates

__ Generalized language is used

__ There is an emphasis on winners and losers

__ There is a cautious atmosphere when issues are discussed

__ Individuals are making efforts to look good

__ *Total Stage II Characteristics*

Stage III: Dysfunctional Patterns Solidify

__ Attempts are made to eliminate others from problem-solving process

__ Obvious leaders or spokespersons have emerged for different sides

__ There is a sense of "holy mission" on the part of certain individuals

__ There is an intention to hurt

__ A choosing up of sides has occurred

__ The leadership good has become identified with a set of special interests

__ There is a sense that the conflict will never end

Continued on next page

<table>
<tr><td>

EXERCISE 6-3 (continued)

__ There has been a loss of middle ground,
with only one-sided, all-or-nothing
options being proposed.

__ *Total Stage III characteristics*

Adapted from: Waitley D. *How to Handle Conflict and Manage Anger: Action Guide.*
Niles, Ill: Nightingale-Conant Corp, 1995. With modifications by Wayne and Mary Sotile,
1998. Used with permission.

Source: Sotile WM, Sotile MO. Conflict management, Part 1: How to shape positive rela-
tionships in medical practices and hospitals. *The Physician Executive.* 999;25(4):57–61.

</td></tr>
</table>

On the other hand, if you are already locked into a Stage III
conflict, you will probably need outside help to resolve your
issues without further damaging your relationship. Consider
seeking professional help from a counselor or consultant trained
in conflict management.

A SYSTEM'S PERSPECTIVE

Conflict is not an individual's problem. Most often, conflict signals a maladaptive relationship or organization. In this sense, two
people engaged in conflict might be symptom bearers of a larger,
dysfunctional work team, hospital community, or family.

Speaking of nonmedical corporate America, anger expert
Hendrie Weisinger[12] delineated a "dirty dozen" list of anger-
provoking work conditions. We have modified Weisinger's
conceptualization to make it relevant to the medical workplace.
We recommend that you periodically review this list to see if
any of these factors apply to your workplace.

What Generates Conflict in the Medical Workplace: The Dirty Dozen and Their Antidotes

1. *General Harassment.* In the medical workplace, we tend to
   think of harassment only happening to nonphysician subordinates. However, physicians complaining of being harassed
   by colleagues, administrators, or an otherwise physician-
   unfriendly work environment is a growing phenomenon.
   Solutions: Appropriate assertiveness, confrontation, limit-
   setting, and negotiation skills

2. *Favoritism.* Even large medical groups tend to be relatively small interpersonal systems. Often, they contain few enough players to allow everyone to know and notice everyone else. Discord can develop when different factions support their cronies when vying for power or influence.

   Solutions: Restore a sense of equity to the situation by operationalizing goals. Accept that not everyone will be equally liked or valued. Distribute leadership responsibilities.

3. *Insensitivity.* Physicians can be blunt in their dealings with each other. Furthermore, many are so guarded against showing vulnerability to their peers that they make it difficult for even their most well-intended colleagues to show sensitivity and concern to them.

   Solutions: If you are a member of an unsupportive organization, take a chance on letting your needs be known. Stay open to supportive interchanges. If things do not change, try to lower your expectations for cordiality and seek support elsewhere. If the insensitivity is abusive, confront the parties involved. If the situation is not corrected, activate your organization's policies and procedures for dealing with such behavior. If this does not help enough, consider whether it is worth it to you to remain in this organization.

4. *Depersonalization.* If physicians begin to feel that they are not valued by the group or organization, conflict is inevitable. Many physicians feel that hospital administrators view them as expendable hired help. Third-party carriers or group administrators interested in filling provider panels with compliant practitioners can overlook years of experience and dedication.

   Solutions: Try to establish genuine relationships. Build a support system and use it to discuss your feelings and experiences. Get involved in extracurricular corporate activities. Assert yourself to get assignments that are meaningful.

5. *Unfair Performance Appraisals.* We have never worked with a "disruptive" physician or a floundering medical student or resident who did not feel unfairly evaluated and labeled by others. High-performing, perfectionistic people do not take kindly to being told that they are not measuring up to someone else's standards.

   Solutions: Try to view criticism as potentially valuable feedback. Concentrate on working to assure that whatever lead to the criticism will not happen again. Avoid showing defensiveness. Increase communication between you and the appraisers. Listen so you can hear the reasons your appraisers are giving you the negative feedback. Ask for specification of what you can do to change the appraisers' perceptions of you.

6. *Lack of Resources.* The ongoing nursing shortage in the United States can seriously strain relationships between physicians and hospital administrators. But limited nursing personnel is not the only potential factor in this category of stressors. Many medical groups progress from being stressed to distressed to demoralized by intragroup disagreement about the optimal number of physicians needed in their organization. In addition, scarcity of resources, like office space, secretarial assistance, research assistants, laboratory services, or prompt and competent consultant services, may also cause distress.

    Solutions: Elicit the cooperation of the gatekeepers to the resources you need. Repeatedly point out what you need and why. Be patient.

7. *Lack of Adequate Training.* One of the most toxic stressors for physicians in training is inadequate supervision. But this stressor is not exclusive to novice physicians. Coping with change requires developing skills that afford reasonable control over the demands created by the change. Here, training in state-of-the art medical technology, information technology, organizational development skills, and emotional management skills all come into play. A variant of this factor occurs when the support personnel you need in order to effectively do your job lack adequate training. Classic here is the situation in which a physician learns a new medical or surgical procedure, but nursing personnel do not. Frustration and added stress—for all parties involved—are sure to result.

    Solutions: If you lack adequate training in a particular area, ask for it or seek it out. If others lack the skills you need for them to have, privately suggest that such training would improve your collaboration. To the extent that you can, offer to help facilitate staff receiving such training.

8. *Lack of Teamwork.* Research has proven that harmonious teamwork promotes stress resilience. "Lone-wolf" players who

refuse to collaborate are sure to prove disruptive to any medical group.

Solutions: Build cooperative relationships. Ask for small favors that you know a coworker is likely to grant. Express appreciation of what others do. Point out how your work affects others and vice versa. Confront colleagues who refuse to cooperate; if they do not respond to all reasonable efforts to improve their collaborative skills, activate your organization's policies and procedures for dealing with individuals who show disruptive workplace behaviors.

9. *Withdrawal of Earned Benefits.* The "double-cross" phenomenon we discussed in Chapter 1 sometimes takes subtle forms. Suffering intangible losses, like loss of autonomy, can be just as demoralizing as more palpable losses, like lost days off, lost benefits, or lost income.

    Solutions: Acknowledge the negative feelings that come in the wake of withdrawal of earned benefits. Specify realistic benefits to be anticipated during a new period of the relationship. Take a leap of faith that the new norm will, indeed, yield the promised benefits. Learn to focus on residual benefits, rather than on what has been lost.

10. *Lack or Violation of Trust.* Again, we harken back to our prior discussion of the "double cross" (Chapter 1). Trust can be damaged in many ways within the medical workplace. Reneged-upon contracts, failure to reciprocate favors like trading on-call responsibilities, disrespectful comments about your competency made in the presence of others—these are but a few of the ways that we have witnessed medical colleagues damaging the trust between themselves and their partners.

    Solutions: Regardless of how it occurs, if your trust is violated, resist the temptation to respond to a trust violation by acting untrustworthy yourself. Accept that trust is a by-product of interpersonal dealings across time and openly state your hope that trust can be rebuilt. Remain aboveboard in your dealings with the other person.

11. *Poor Communication.* Many of the factors in this "dirty dozen" list are caused or complicated by poor communication. The intensity and diversity inherent in working in medicine can

make effective communication with others a difficult goal to achieve.

Solutions: With regularity, accurately identify and appropriately express what you think, feel, need, and want in your relationships.

12. *An Incompetent Superior.* The range of experience and expertise within any group of medical peers tends to be wide. Younger physicians may feel that their senior colleagues, although clearly more experienced, are not as well trained as they are. Partners in a group practice may doubt the business savvy or administrative skills of the very colleagues they elected to head their organization. And junior faculty may question the competency of their Chair or of their institution's administration. In either case, tensions result.

Solutions: Claim responsibility and authority where possible. Push for management by committee. Stay focused on your own work and duties, rather than on the behavior of others.

WHAT YOU CAN DO TO CORRECT OR PREVENT CONFLICT

This entire chapter addresses various ways to correct or prevent conflict in the workplace. Here, we emphasize one key concept and one strategy that should always be included in your organization's culture.

Accept That Disagreements Will Inevitably Occur

Effective conflict management starts with a realistic attitude about relationship dynamics. In truth, whenever two or more people gather for any length of time, disagreement will eventually occur. The crucial action involves what happens *next*. How you react to your disagreements—and not whether or not you disagree—will determine the quality of your relationship. Preventing the development of conflict requires that you maturely accept the fact that, for the duration of this relationship, you will have to periodically and repeatedly work to resolve disagreements.

Regularly Get and Give 360 Degree Feedback

EEM requires a regular, honest assessment of your relationships. Often, feedback from others helps. Feedback may be delivered in many ways, including family counseling sessions, self-observational exercises, coaching, counseling, formal psychological testing, or peer ratings in the medical workplace. Seeing yourself through the eyes of others can sharpen your vision—and heighten your humility—regarding your interpersonal style. And reflective self-awareness can empower you.

Research in the corporate workplace has proven this last point. Receiving feedback that allows you to see yourself through the eyes of others has been shown to improve interpersonal effectiveness and mitigate the deleterious effects of stress, burnout, and impairment.[13] Other studies[14,15] have demonstrated that as managers develop insight into their own behaviors based on reviews from peers, ratings of their managerial performance by subordinates, peers, and supervisors improves.[14,15]

A process used by management consultants can provide the kinds of insights that were found to be so powerful in these studies. A "360° feedback" requires that every member of an organization or work team offers both positive and negative feedback to every other member. The feedback focuses on what it is like to work with the targeted individual. In our consultation with medical practices, we have found the simple evaluation form shown in Figure 6-1 to be quite useful in providing such feedback.[16]

It is imperative to use this or any feedback process in a constructive manner. Medical workplaces would do well to adopt the ethic espoused by other corporate cultures: Feedback is not a form of "witch hunting;" it is essential to ongoing efforts for continuous improvement in the work team.

And remember: Leaders go first. Volunteering to be the first target of such feedback is a helpful way to sell the idea to your group and to hone your own leadership skills.

F I G U R E   6-1

Feedback Form

Physician to be Evaluated:_____

Please indicate how often the physician named above exhibits the behavior described in each of the numbered items below. Use the back of this sheet for additional comments. Thank you.

	Never	Rarely	Sometimes	Often
1. Is a clear communicator.				
2. Accepts constructive criticism.				
3. Staff complain of his/her behavior.				
4. Patients complain of his/her behavior.				
5. Is trustworthy.				
6. Is reasonably courteous to me when we work together.				
7. Puts self-interests before group interests.				
8. Works hard for the betterment of the group.				
9. Responds to pages in a timely, courteous fashion.				
10. Offers constructive input during staff meetings.				
11. Tries to sidestep rules.				
12. Shames others for negative outcomes.				
13. Threatens retribution or litigation.				
14. Uses foul language, shouting, or rudeness.				
15. Lets me know that what I contribute to the group is appreciated.				

Your name:_____Date:_____

Please indicate below what you appreciate or admire about this physician:

_____

Additional comments:

_____

Thank you.

CONCLUSIONS

EEM requires that you develop sophisticated skills for managing relationship dynamics. Identifying your personal conflict management style and factors that might impede your progress when negotiating conflict is an important starting point. However, diagnosis is not enough. You must also commit yourself to learning the skills needed to be interpersonally *effective*. Our next two chapters outline the skills needed for just such effectiveness.

REFERENCES–CHAPTER 6

1. Goleman D. *Emotional Intelligence.* New York, NY: Bantam; 1995.
2. Weber DO. Cooling it gets hot. *The Physician Executive.* 1999;25:8–14.
3. Aschenbrener CA, Siders CT. Managing low-to-mid intensity conflict in the health care setting. *The Physician Executive.* 1999;25:44–50.
4. Arnetz BB. White collar stress: What studies of physicians can teach us. *Psychother Psychosom.* 1991;55:197–200.
5. Silverman MM. Physicians and suicide. In: Goldman LS, Myers M, Dickstein LJ, eds. *The Handbook of Physician Health.* Chicago, Ill: American Medical Association; 2000:95–117.
6. Kilmann RH, Thomas KW. Developing a forced-choice measure of conflict-handling behavior: The "mode" instrument. *Educ Psycholog Dev.* 1977;37:309–325.
7. Waitley D. *Anger management tapes. How to handle conflict and manage anger: Action guide.* Niles, Ill: Nightingale-Conant Corp; 1995.
8. Sotile WM, Sotile MO. The angry physician: The temper-tantruming physician. *The Physician Executive.* 1996;22:30–34.
9. Sotile WM, Sotile. MO. Conflict management, Part 1: How to shape positive relationships in medical practices and hospitals. *The Physician Executive.* 1999;25:57–61.
10. Dawson R, Why do physicians have difficulty negotiating? *The Physician Executive.* 1999;25:43–44.
11. Babitsky S, Mangraviti JJ. *The Successful Physician Negotiator: How to Get What You Deserve.* Falmouth, Mass: SEAK, Inc; 1998.
12. Weisinger H. *Anger at Work.* New York: William Morrow and Co; 1995.
13. Kilburg RR. *Executive Coaching: Developing Managerial Wisdom in a World of Chaos.* Washington, DC: American Psychological Association; 2000.
14. Church AH. Managerial self-awareness in high-performing individuals in organizations. *J Appl Psychol.* 1997;87:281–292.
15. Yammarino FJ, Atwater LE. Understanding self-perception accuracy: Implications for human resource management. *Hum Res Manage.* 1993;32(2-3):231–247.
16. Pfifferling JH. Managing the unmanageable: The disruptive physician. *Fam Pract Manage.* Nov/Dec,1997:77–92.

c h a p t e r | 7

Anger Management

"Anger has the capacity to be the good, the bad, and the ugly. It is up to each of us to maximize its good, minimize the bad, and eliminate the ugly."

> Hendrie Weisenger, PhD
> *Anger at Work*[1]

Scene 1:

> *Nurse:* "Dr Jones, I'm sorry to wake you, but I thought you should know that Ms. Johnson is in tremendous pain and her surgical wound is inflamed and oozing."
>
> *Dr Jones:* (irritated) "Did you even read the chart note that I left this evening, instructing you what to do in case this happened?"
>
> *Nurse:* "Yes I did. And I'm sorry to have to call. But I was not quite sure about this."
>
> *Dr Jones:* (sarcastically) "You people are never 'quite sure' about anything. Why can't we get competent nurses in this hospital? (angrily) I swear, I am fed up with your inappropriate calls. You shouldn't be working in a hospital if you aren't smart enough to read and follow directions."

Scene 2:

> *Wife:* (shouting) "I'm sick and tired of this! You are never supportive when I need you to be."
>
> *Husband:* (angrily) "Why don't you just quiet down and act like you've got good sense."
>
> *Wife:* "I'll show you how good my sense is. I'll leave you, and then let's see how you get along."
>
> *Husband:* "Why don't you shut up, stop threatening, and do something other than whine and complain all the time."
>
> *Wife:* "I should never have married you in the first place."

How does a caring, competent person end up abdicating control of his or her own behavior to the extent depicted in each of the preceding examples? What causes these sorts of internal and behavioral storms? What can be done about it?

According to behavioral health experts, anger is the mood people are worst at controlling.[2] (Sadness, on the other hand, is the mood people put most effort into shaking.) Whether in the form of amygdala-driven sparks of rage at injustice and unfairness or the neocortex-driven anger expressed in calculated, cool-headed acts of revenge, poorly managed anger hurts stress hardiness.

In this chapter, we discuss the causes and consequences of and solutions to mismanaged anger. We describe a step-by-step process that can help you to develop healthy ways of coping with anger.

UNDERSTANDING THE PHENOMENOLOGY OF AN ANGER OUTBURST

The universal trigger for anger is a sense of being endangered. This may come in the form of a physical threat. More often, though, anger is stirred by symbolic threats to one's self-esteem or dignity, being treated unjustly or rudely, being insulted or demeaned, or being frustrated in pursuing an important goal.[3]

Stress of all sorts lowers the threshold for anger. Given the stresses and frustrations inherent in a life in medicine, learning to manage anger is a survival skill necessary to construct a successful personal and professional life.

Psychologist Gerald Patterson[4] pointed out that escalating anger depends on chains of interactions in which two people attempt to influence each other through a rapid exchange of punishing communications. Escalating aversive chains are especially likely to occur between two people of approximately equal power: husband/wife, colleagues in the workplace, or parents/ children (equal because both parties are emotionally vulnerable to the other).

These aversive chains tend to progress through predictable stages. Irritable exchanges at first appear trivial and therefore are overlooked. Back-and-forth jibes or hostile remarks that go on for three or four steps within a 30-second period of time are not

F I G U R E   7-1

An Anger Sequence

Event → physiological arousal → angry thoughts → emotional arousal → sarcastic or otherwise critical behavior → further emotional and physiological arousal → further angry thoughts → increased tension → aggressive behavior → eventual withdrawal from others → thoughts that fuel further resentment and physiological arousal → re-engagement with irritable, abrupt tones → defensiveness → argumentativeness → disengagement[8]

uncommon in strained relationships. Most people stop interacting at that point, go their separate ways, and things cool down.

But if one or both individuals refuse to disengage and, instead, continue to badger, defend, and counterattack, interactions are likely to heat up to the point of incorporating threats and/or physical violence. The last link in the chain that precedes or precipitates a violent outburst is termed "trigger behavior." These can be verbal or nonverbal behaviors that stir in others feelings like abandonment, rejection, disrespect, or alarm. Frequently, an anger sequence involves the building blocks depicted in Figure 7-1.

DOES EXPRESSING ANGER ALWAYS HURT?

Expressing anger can be a healthy choice. Anger helps us to defend ourselves if we are physically threatened, if our boundaries are being violated, or if we need help to overcome our fears.[5] "Without anger, problems go unnoticed, situations become worse, injustice and abuse run rampant."[1 (p. 165)]

Anger management experts generally agree that venting anger does not dispel it.[6] Lashing out and venting does have some momentary benefits *if* done under certain conditions like the following:

- If expressed directly to the person who is the true target
- When doing so restores a sense of control
- When it rights an injustice
- When it inflicts "appropriate harm" on the other person and gets him to change some grievous activity without retaliating[7]

But the "anger habit" can be rather addictive. Studies have shown that verbal and physical expression of anger lowers the threshold of acting that way again.[8]

Far more often, expressing anger creates or complicates problems. First, if you mismanage anger, you will lose your ability to effectively deal with others. As we mentioned earlier, high-powered people often live in a surprising paradox: Despite their intimidating style, they secretly feel helpless and vulnerable in relationships. Typically, their aggressiveness and defensiveness have to do with deeply felt anxieties and insecurities about their own worth and about their ability to deal with others.[9] But their behavior complicates, rather than soothes, their tensions.[10] Research has clearly shown that if you justify unbridled outbursts of anger with the notion that it's better to express anger than it is to hold it inside, you are making a serious mistake. The truth is that aggressive behavior simply begets more aggression on the parts of both parties.[11]

Mismanaged anger also blunts our awareness. Many high-performing people learn "feeling substitutions" like the following: It's not okay to feel vulnerable emotions like anxiety, fear, disappointment, depression, hurt, guilt, shame, or failure; *but it is okay to feel angry*; It's not okay to feel painful sensations like fatigue, physical pain, or overstimulation; *but it is okay to feel angry*; It's not okay to feel positive feelings like warmth, intimacy, neediness, or succorance; *but it is okay to feel angry*.

Like one-trick ponies, such people go through life showing anger no matter what they feel. The result? They fail to accurately communicate their needs to others and their relationships prove to be more stressful than soothing.

Anger also affects our thinking. High levels of rage lead to cognitive incapacitation during which the person dismisses mitigating information. Because a bout of anger involves a cognitive shift into selectively perceiving negatives and rigidly treating assumptions as though they were facts, anger diminishes our more adaptive cognitive processes, such as memory, creativity, and concentration.[1] Rigid, angry thinking blots out our ability to effectively problem-solve and to self-soothe in adaptive ways.

Mismanaged hostility is also one of the most dangerous risks to your health. Hostility researchers Redford and Virginia Williams warn that for the chronically hostile person, "getting angry is like taking a small dose of some slow-acting poison—arsenic, for example—every day of your life."[8] Furthermore, research has shown that low serotonin levels correlate with increased depression and increased levels of aggressive, violent behavior problems.[8,12] The serotonin-enhancing drug Prozac, on the other hand, decreased aggressive behavior and increased affiliative behavior in monkeys.[13] Our clinical experiences certainly attest to the benefits of incorporating the use of antidepressant medications into the treatment of chronically hostile individuals.

HOW TO TAKE CONTROL OF YOUR ANGRY REACTIONS

Our anger management counseling with physicians follows this six-step approach:

1. Identify the three "flavors" of angry reactions.
2. Pinpoint what your anger is about.
3. Be honest about the effects of your anger.
4. Learn to accurately identify when you are angry versus when you are otherwise physiologically "activated" or "aroused."
5. Disrupt anger-generating sequences, including the thoughts and behaviors that perpetuate anger.
6. Use response rehearsal and mental imagery to internalize new anger management strategies.

Each step is elaborated in the following paragraphs.

The Three Flavors of Anger

Managing anger starts with recognizing that what we typically refer to simply as "anger" actually involves three distinct phenomena. Health psychologist Timothy Smith of the University of Utah[14] reminded us that *anger* is an unpleasant *emotional experience* that may range from irritation to rage. *Hostility,* on the other hand, is a set of *negative attitudes or beliefs* that others will probably mistreat, frustrate, or provoke you and therefore are not to be trusted.

Finally, there is *aggression*—overt *behavior* that typically involves attacking, destructive, or hurtful actions. The three flavors of anger interrelate: If you get stuck in the habit of being angry, the odds increase that you will develop hostile, cynical attitudes that will lead you to act unnecessarily aggressive.

Learn What Your Anger is About

In prior work,[15] we pointed out that chronically angry people tend to show some combination of three syndromes:

- Anger signals ongoing struggle with some disappointment or loss from the past.
- Anger flares because you are dissatisfied with some major aspect of your present life.
- Anger is the by-product of your personality-based coping patterns.

Disappointments and Losses

Experiencing loss is an unavoidable part of living. Many folks get stuck in the angry stage of grief over losses. The questions here are: What losses have you experienced that have been particularly difficult to endure and how are you currently coping with these?

As you examine these questions, you may be saddened to realize just how much you have lost during your life. Included here are the obvious losses: deaths of loved ones or friends, lost friendships, health problems, or failures. These dramatic losses are typically identified and openly grieved, and acknowledging them usually leads to support, relief, and healing.

But most of us also suffer various "disenfranchised" losses—those that are not typically recognized and expressed and therefore tend not to heal. Included here are more subtle losses such as: loss of your youth, loss of valued opportunities like spending more time with your family when you and they were younger, loss of dreams that did not come true, loss of the ways it used to be during simpler times, or loss of fun and passion in some areas of your life like your work.

Health care professionals are especially prone to accumulate unresolved grief over the deaths of patients. Unfortunately, the world does not recognize physician grief. When was the last time anyone expressed sympathy or offered you special, nurturing care when one of your patients died? To the contrary, we have heard brutal, traumatizing stories from physicians who were openly blamed and shamed by superiors or aggrieved loved ones after the death of a patient.

When we do not openly or fully grieve, we get stuck in some painful emotion at some point in the fairly predictable stages of grief. Furthermore, we believe that grieving major losses typically unfolds over years, not months. Anyone who loses a cherished loved one knows how true this is. Just because loss occurred in the distant past, don't assume that your grieving is necessarily finished.

If your anger signals unfinished grieving, then you must allow yourself to complete the process. This means finding a safe relationship in which you can talk about what you are feeling. Expressing painful emotions and getting support not only lessens grief, it also prevents the physical complications to health that can come from suppressing negative emotions.

Let yourself feel and talk about your losses. You might find it helpful to write out your feelings, expressing what you appreciated and regretted about the relationship, person, or situation that you lost. Remember: Grief is an emotional process that dissipates if it is fully experienced. Don't be afraid of your painful emotions. With the support of others and with a nurturing and self-accepting attitude, let yourself grieve until you are relieved.

Maybe I'm Just Not Satisfied

Anger does not always have to do with grief over what is past. For some, anger comes from their here-and-now struggles—something about the situations, relationships, or processes that create their life territory is toxic.

One obvious way to lessen your anger is to create a life territory that is more to your liking. This may mean finding the courage to change where you live, how you live, or with whom you deal. Eliminating toxic situations, processes, or people from your life is not necessarily the same as running from your problems. More often, it's about defending your right to live a more healthy, meaningful life.

Of course, this is not always possible. Some stresses can't be eliminated. You may suffer from something (such as an illness) or from some relationship (such as with one of your loved ones) that is not changeable. In these circumstances, rather than changing the *external* causes of your anger, you must learn to change your *internal* reactions. This involves taking an honest look at how your personality drives you into anger.

TABLE   7-1

Personality Drivers and Anger

If your personality compels you to:	You will likely experience anger in the following situations:
Be Strong	When you are challenged, during interpersonal conflict, or when you are asked to talk about your inner thoughts or feelings.
Be Perfect	When your quests for perfection are encumbered by your own or another's lack of perfection or when you perceive someone as challenging your control.
Please Others	When you are accused of behaving selfishly.
Try Hard	When you are accused of being lazy or of not having tried hard enough or when you deal with others who do not seem to share your value for hard work.
Hurry Up	When you are forced to slow your urgent pace because of some unexpected factor such as someone else moving slowly or due to your own limitations.
Be Careful	When you are asked to trust that another will be competent or nurturing.

Source: Sotile WM, Sotile MO. *The Medical Marriage: Sustaining Healthy Relationships for Physicians and Their Families.* Chicago, Ill: American Medical Association; 2000.

Personality Scripting

Certain situations are especially likely to stir anger for people driven by each of the personality scripts referred to earlier. Review Table 7-1 and note what applies to you.

Once you identify the sorts of situations that are most likely to stir your anger, beware. Accept that some of these situations are probably inevitable parts of your life, and remind yourself to take extra care to remain mindful of your thoughts and behaviors during these circumstances.

Regardless of its cause and your level of justification about being angry, the question is one of pragmatics. Is your way of managing your anger wreaking havoc on your life? To answer this important question, complete Exercise 7-1.

How Is Your Anger Affecting Your Life?

What toll is your anger taking on your body and your relationships? In *When Anger Hurts: Quieting the Storm Within,*[5] authors

E X E R C I S E   7-1

Anger Impact Inventory

0 = No Effect   1 = Minor Effect   2 = Moderate Effect
3 = Very Significant Effect   4 = Major Effect

Instructions: Using the five-point rating scale, rate the degree of impact your anger has on the following:

                                                                          Rating

1. Relationships to authorities   ____

2. Relationships to peers and colleagues at work   ____

3. Relationships to subordinates at work   ____

4. Relationships to patients   ____

5. Relationships to hospital administrators   ____

6. Relationships to children   ____

7. Relationships to children's teachers and other parents   ____

8. Relationships to spouse or lover   ____

9. Relationships to previous spouse or lover   ____

10. Relationships to parents   ____

11. Relationships to other family members   ____

12. Relationships to current friends   ____

13. Relationships to former friends   ____

14. Relationships to neighbors   ____

15. Relationships to recreational groups or organizations   ____

16. Relationships to political and other groups   ____

17. Your health   ____

18. Physical symptoms (rapid heart rate, tension, shoulder and neck
    pain, headache, irritability, feeling of pressure, restlessness,
    insomnia, brooding, and so on)   ____

19. Productivity   ____

20. Relaxation or pleasurable activities (sex, sports, hobbies, and so on) ____

21. Drinking or drug use   ____

22. Creativity   ____

23. Driving   ____

24. Accidents   ____

25. Work-related errors and mistakes   ____

26. Collegiality   ____

Source: McKay M, Rogers PD, McKay J. *When Anger Hurts: Quieting the Storm Within.* Oakland, Calif: New Harbinger Press, 1989. Modified with permission.

Matthew and Judith McKay and Peter Rogers present the "Anger Impact Inventory," a tool that can help you assess the costs of your anger. In Exercise 7-1, we have modified this instrument to make it applicable to physicians.

McKay and colleagues[5] recommend that you analyze your responses to see if any patterns emerge. Are you angrier at home or at work? Do you tend to feel angrier with certain people or in certain situations? Are a significant number of your relationships contaminated by your anger? Now is the time to identify one or two areas in which you are willing to concentrate your efforts to improve.

Learn to Notice When You are Angry Versus Physiologically Aroused

As we have mentioned several times, pattern disruption is a key to EES. Keeping an anger journal can facilitate the disruption of anger reactions.[5] Periodically throughout the day, say once every 2 hours, chart the number of times you got angry since your last journal entry. Next, rate how aroused you feel at this moment. Try to differentiate *physiological arousal* (eg, signs of the fight-or-flight syndrome, such as rapid heart rate, shallow breathing, muscular tension, and so forth) from *emotional arousal* (eg, how angry you feel). Use a scale of 1 to 10, with 1 = minimal arousal and 10 = worst anger arousal ever.

This exercise can benefit you in several ways. First, it is important to learn to recognize states of both types of arousal. Classically, high-anger people find themselves in some variant of the following conversation:

> *Person 1:* "You don't have to get so angry! Stop yelling at me."
> *Person 2:* "I'm not yelling, and I'm not angry. I'm just trying to get you to listen to me!"
> *Person 1:* "You *are* yelling, and you obviously *are* angry."

Many of our patients have gained great insight from simply learning to differentiate arousal from anger. Physiological activation does not have to lead to an angry episode. Learning to recognize when you are alarmed, frightened, challenged, excited, or otherwise activated can help you to avoid simply acting angry, even when you are not.

If your journal entry indicates that, indeed, you *are* angry, your task is to analyze your current angry state and develop a plan of action for managing it. Start by noting what event or events stirred your anger. If there are no clear causes of your irritability, note what may have stressed you during the preceding block of time. Ask, "What was I feeling before I got angry? Am I blocking or displacing some feeling or stress by being angry?"

Also, take time to analyze your anger journal entries. Novack and coworkers,[16] discussing patient–physician interactions, suggested a series of self-examination questions that can help you to take responsibility for your part of patient–physician relationships. We modified these to apply to any relationship:

- What sorts of (people) elicit an angry reaction in me?
- What work situation usually makes me angry and why?
- What are my usual responses to my own anger and the anger of others? (eg, Do I overreact, placate, blame others, suppress my own feelings, become superreasonable?)
- What are the underlying feelings when I become angry (eg, feeling rejected, humiliated, unworthy)?
- Where did I learn my responses to anger?
- How might I be relating my family roles to my roles in my work environment?
- What lessons did I learn from my family about the nature of relationships, about the nature of caregiving, and about acceptable responses to conflict?
- What types of colleagues might I be likely to associate with family members?

Disrupt Anger Sequences

Keeping an anger journal is a step toward awareness, and awareness leads to control. As you begin to see how often you are experiencing feelings of anger, you can begin to change the unproductive behavioral sequences you may have become accustomed to. Disrupting these sequences requires four steps:

1. Identify provocations and develop a plan.
2. Counter physiological arousal.
3. Control anger thinking.
4. Control your behavior.

Step 1. Identify Provocations and Develop a Plan
The information from your anger journal can help you to better prepare for dealing with situations or people that carry a high risk of stirring your anger. It is best to prepare when you are in a low degree of anger arousal. Once you are angry, it is difficult to accurately analyze your options.

This caveat notwithstanding, it is still important to get inquisitive rather than aggressive or presumptive when you are angry. Learn to let being angry automatically stir your inquisitiveness. Anger management experts[1,8] emphasize that asking yourself a series of questions like those listed below can help you to at once identify provocations and begin to take control of your reactions.

- That's interesting: I'm feeling angry. Now what might this be about?
- Have I stumbled into one of the high-risk situations that I know from past experience tend to "hook" me?
- Is this really how I want to be feeling right now?
- Is there anything specific that is really triggering my anger? If so, what is it? If not, what might I be able to do *right now* that might help me to distract myself and calm down?

Step 2. Counter Physiological Arousal
The physiological correlates of a bout of anger include elevated levels of testosterone, cortisol, epinephrine, and norepinephrine. Typically, the sympathetic activation that comes with anger is followed by a burst of acetylcholine, which turns off the harsh effects of adrenaline and other substances produced by the sympathetic nervous system when you are angry. But some hot reactors have underactive parasympathetic calming responses.[8]

A key to anger management is to learn to recognize signs of physiological arousal and to learn to use these as a signal that it is time for you to generate different types of cognitive, behavioral, and physical responses so that your arousal does not turn into anger. Anger management experts[1,5,8] recommend that you learn to convert the physical arousal into a form of energy that gives you the impetus to confront your provocations effectively.

This is most effectively done if you can learn to do two things. First, you must learn to discriminate your various "flavors" of arousal. This is easier said than done, given that, from a physiological perspective, many different experiences have similar physical manifestations. For example, your body responds similarly to feeling rushed, frustrated, irritated, sexually aroused, angry, frightened, embarrassed, challenged, or excited. To discern the emotion that you are feeling during such states of arousal requires that you slow your pace, focus your attention inward, and be honest about what you think and feel at the moment.

The second strategy for countering physiology that may fuel anger reactions is to generate alternative states of arousal when you are getting angry. These might include moments of relaxation, humor, affection, compassion, empathy, inquisitiveness, or spiritual connection with your Higher Power. Any of these experiences tends to release endorphins that calm otherwise stormy physiology.

Step 3. Manage Anger-Generating Thoughts

Certain kinds of thinking seem to inevitably correlate with periods of anger arousal. Psychologist Robert Alan[17] emphasizes that anger often signals a threat to an underlying need and occurs as a result of what he calls an anger-judgment complex whereby anger is fueled either by the judgment that you are being done an injustice or the judgment that your stress is happening due to someone's incompetence. *A judgment of injustice* might involve seeing the situation that you face as being unfair, improper, wrong, or the result of someone being inconsiderate or biased in dealing with you. *A judgment of incompetence* might involve seeing your stress as being caused by another's shortcomings, such as their stupidity, laziness, inadequacy, or lack of qualifications.

Hendrie Weisenger[1] pointed out that we tend to think anger-generating thoughts, not only when we perceive that others did not do what they "ought to" have done but when we violate our own usually inflated self-expectations. At such times, we are especially prone to distorted thinking like magnifying blemishes and minimizing what is right about the situation, person, or oneself; destructive labeling that stirs malevolent feelings toward others or oneself; or mind reading that results in assumptions of "worst-case" scenarios.

One way to counter anger-generating judgments is to charitably put yourself in the other person's place. Develop the habit of reminding yourself that others are doing the best they can to cope with their world, given who they are and what they have learned from their own experiences.

For example, let's say that you are stuck in a slow-moving checkout line in a grocery store. You notice that the cashier seems to be taking her time in checking out each customer. She moves slowly, chats with each customer, and generally seems to be in no particular hurry to move the line along.

Your reflexive reaction to this situation might be anger-fueling thoughts such as:

"This jerk could care less how long she takes to check us out! Just because she has this dead-head job, she probably thinks that the rest of us have nothing better to do than to stand here and take her foolishness. I swear, I'm sick and tired of taking this kind of foolishness from people!"

Notice that these thoughts are filled with judgments. They suggest that the checkout clerk is purposely persecuting the customers with her incompetence and with her lackadaisical attitude.

A more empathic and self-controlled way of reacting to the same situation might be:

"This line is not moving! That checkout clerk is a slow worker. This aggravates me.

Okay. Now, let's see. I *am* angry, but I guess I *do* have a choice about how I think and act right now. I could decide that this young woman is doing the best that she can. Maybe she's just a hard-working kid who is not very bright. Maybe she's just trying to learn how to be a good worker. We all had to start someplace. I can appreciate that; I remember how I fumbled through my first job.

I might as well find a way to enjoy myself as much as I can while I wait. Maybe I'll use this time to practice relaxing. Maybe I'll just read one of these junk tabloids that I don't usually buy. Maybe I'll just have a nice vacation fantasy."

Use the list of self-statements in Table 7-2 to help control your internal responses during frustrating situations.[18] See such situations as opportunities to practice anger control. Remind yourself that developing the habit of reacting to others with empathy rather than criticism will serve you well.

Step 4. Control Your Behaviors

The next step in managing anger is not psychological; it's behavioral. Even if you seem unable to control your thinking and if your anger is flowing, you will preserve your health and your relationships if you block your urge to act aggressively. This is not only tactful, it is wise. The aforementioned health risks of chronic

T A B L E 7-2

Managing Anger: Coping Statements

"No point in blaming. I'll try a new strategy."

"I may not like it, but he/she is probably doing his/her best right now."

"I have a choice about how I react right now."

"Is this worth dying for?"

"Will this matter 5 years from now?"

"If I am still angry about this tomorrow, I'll deal with it then."

"I am free to want what I want, but he or she is free to be different from me."

"I am not in charge of the world."

"Anger will not get me what I want."

"Acting angry is not the same as showing that I care."

"Calmness is not the same as weakness."

"There is power in calmness."

"It's time to relax."

"Let me ask, rather than tell."

"I'll listen, rather than talk."

"This is interesting; let me try to figure it out."

"I can feel strongly and act calmly."

"Remember to laugh."

"I'm in charge of how I react, not him/her."

"How big is this issue, compared to the size of my life?"

"Being in a hurry just makes me irritable and not nice to be around."

"I deserve to enjoy."

"Hostility is bad for my health."

"My need to control others is fueled by my own insecurities."

"It takes real strength and maturity to show love and kindness."

"This is just a drop of water in a waterfall."

Source: Sotile WM. *Heart Illness and Intimacy: How Caring Relationships Aid Recovery.* Baltimore, Md: Johns Hopkins University Press, 1992. Used with permission.

hostility are attenuated if aggression is tempered. That means that even if you cannot manage your angry emotions or your hostile thoughts, you can keep from doing harm to yourself and to others if you learn to behave in ways that are not aggressive. For example, researchers have found that modifying your style of speech when having a conflict lessens strain on your heart, even if you are highly angry or frustrated during the conflict.[19]

TABLE 7-3

Ways to Fuel Anger

General Category	Specific Examples
Verbal Behaviors	Cursing
	Giving unwanted advice
	Criticizing
	Threatening
	Blaming
	Exaggerating
	Giving ultimatums
	Being sarcastic
	Refusing to discuss the topic
Nonverbal Sounds	Sighing
	Moaning
	Grunting
	Groaning
Voice Quality, Tone, and Volume	Shouting
	Tense, overly controlled
	Mumbling
	Snickering
	Whining
	Flatness, suggesting disinterest
Hand and Arm Gestures	Balling fist
	Pointing a finger
	Shaking a fist
	Folding arms
	Placing hands on hips
	Waving hand, suggesting dismissal
	Pounding or tapping table
	Chopping motion
Facial Expressions	Rolling eyes
	Refusal to make eye contact
	Narrowing eyes
	Grimacing in disgust or disbelief
	Raising eyebrows
	Frowning
	Scowling
Body Movements	Shaking head, indicating "No, no!"
	Shrugging shoulders
	Foot tapping
	Turning away
	Pacing
	Kicking
	Pushing or grabbing

Source: McKay M, Rogers PD, McKay J. *When Anger Hurts: Quieting the Storm Within.* Oakland, Calif: New Harbinger Press, 1989. Modified with permission.

We have worked with countless high-powered people who have benefited markedly from simply learning to differentiate assertion from aggression. In doing so, they have reclaimed their personal power and control in their dealings with difficult people and difficult situations. This requires that you pay particular attention to six aspects of your communication style.[5] These are your: verbal behaviors; nonverbal sounds; voice quality, tone, and volume; hand and arm gestures; facial expressions; and body movements. Table 7-3 lists anger-fueling mistakes to be avoided in each of these six categories.

Unfortunately, once we are angry, most of us lose sight of our actions and the impact we are having on others. Often, we express anger in ways that simply perpetuate angry reactions from others, and our own anger reactions escalate. Listening to an audiotape or watching a video of yourself as you deal with a frustrating situation can be an invaluable, sobering experience. This is what happened to Charles when he watched a video replay of a family therapy session in which he angrily criticized his wife and son. "I got scared looking at myself on that tape," he said sadly. "No wonder my family avoids me whenever things get tense!"

Anger Generators and Minimizers

How you behave when you are angry sets the tone of your interactions with others that will then either fuel your anger or calm you. Use the "Angry Behaviors Scale" in Exercise 7-2 to assess whether you tend to generate or minimize anger behaviors.

A number of strategies for better controlling anger can be gleaned from the above information. First, analyze the information in the "Ways to Fuel Anger" table and the "Angry Behaviors" scale. Ask loved ones and colleagues or staff members for feedback about your style of communicating during disagreements. Try not to get defensive when hearing this feedback. The purpose here is not to start another argument; we simply want you to develop a realistic picture of yourself. You can then use this picture as a guideline for changing.

Next comes the hard part: *You must practice reacting differently.* Once again, review the tables in this chapter, this time taking note of alternatives to ineffectual behaviors in each of the major categories. Then practice these more controlled ways of acting. Periodically tape-record your conversations with your staff or

E X E R C I S E   7-2

Angry Behaviors Scale

Rate yourself on each behavioral dimension by placing an "X" nearest the description of your most typical interpersonal behavior.

Anger Generators   **Anger Minimizers**

Use disrespectful tones or behaviors_____Show respect

Don't look at the other person_____Make eye contact

Make unreasonable demands_____Focus on practical solutions

Act like I need to be right_____Keep an open mind

Pass judgments_____Suspend judgments

Sarcasm, humiliation, attacks, threats_____Even, calm, but firm tone

Touch or get too close_____Maintain appropriate distance

Use aggressive gestures_____Use neutral, open gestures

Send mixed messages_____Send consistent messages

Show favoritism_____ Act fairly

Show impatience or act bored_____Use active listening skills

Act inflexibly_____Act flexibly

Interrupt_____Allow reasonable venting

Use negative words_____Use positive phrases

Reject the person_____Focus on behaviors

Constantly override decisions_____Encourage collaboration

Fail to follow through_____Follow through on promises

Lie_____Be honest

Don't respond to individual needs_____Treat others as individuals

Source: Modified from: Staver, M. *21 Ways to Diffuse Anger and Calm People Down.* Boulder, Colo: CareerTrack Pub; 1995. Used with permission.

family and then review the tape to listen for changes in
your style.

Finally, we recommend that you explicitly state your commitment to learn to negotiate your differences without damaging your
relationship. It is never too late to benefit from positive change. If
you sincerely apologize for past, inappropriate behavior, commit
yourself to changing, and, indeed, follow through, you can generate
new levels of trust, self-respect, and healthy relationships.

Slow Down and/or Call Time Out

When things get tense, it is crucial to resist the temptation to
speed up and intensify your interactions. Instead, first try to slow
down the process. McKay and collegues[5] recommend that you
learn to automatically use the following five lines when things
get tense:

- I'm feeling (state what's bothering you). And what I think I
  need (want or would like) in this situation is . . .
- What would you propose to solve this problem?
- If (the problem) goes on, I'll have to (a self-care solution) in
  order to take care of myself.
- What do you need in this situation? (Concerns, worries you)
  (bothering you?)
- So what you want is . . .

If need be, call a time-out from a heated interaction. This can be
an effective way to disrupt anger swirls. Doing so allows you to
calm activated physiology, collect your thoughts, and develop a
new and more helpful perspective on how to deal with the problem and the person you are having conflict with. You can call
time-out with a simple statement like this: "I'm feeling pretty
stressed. I want to stop and cool off for a while."

If you do call time-out, be sure to use the pause appropriately.
Do something to healthily release tension. Avoid caffeine or stimulating drugs or alcohol and any agitating behaviors, like driving.
Don't hang onto angry thoughts during your time-out. Instead,
try to relax and clear your mind. After an appropriate time (we
recommend at least 30 minutes), take responsibility for reinitiat-
ing the conversation with the other person.

USE RESPONSE REHEARSAL AND MENTAL IMAGERY

If you can imagine it, you can "pretend" it. If you "pretend" it long enough, you become it. This adage from cognitive/behavioral therapy highlights the importance of using mental rehearsal and behavioral follow-through in changing old habits. Take time to picture yourself managing anger appropriately. Imagine upcoming meetings or conversations and see, feel, and hear yourself responding in a way that demonstrates effective, assertive anger management. This form of mental rehearsal will help to counter otherwise destructive, anger-generating ways of thinking as you prepare for an already stressful event. Mental rehearsal also serves to remind you of the many strategies for effective anger control you have at your disposal.

CONCLUSIONS

The stresses of a busy life inevitably create periods of irritation and anger. How you manage these emotions will shape your relationships and affect your quality of life, both at home and work.

We do not mean to imply that resilient physicians are always mellow. To do so would be to create a false standard of mental health. But this is clear: Physicians today cannot afford mismanaged anger. Indeed, emotions are contagious, and how you manage anger will shape relationship dynamics that will either bless or stress you and those around you.

Geared with the tools needed to manage yourself, you are now ready to address how you might go about managing others when they are upset. We address this important topic in our next two chapters.

REFERENCES–CHAPTER 7

1. Weisenger H. *Anger at Work.* New York, NY: William Morrow and Co; 1995.

2. Tice D, Baumeister RF. Controlling anger: Self-induced emotional change. In: Wenger D, Pennebaker J, eds. *Handbook of Mental Control,* vol. 5. Englewood Cliffs, NJ: Prentice-Hall; 1993.

3. Zillmann D. Mental control of angry aggression. In: Wegner D, Pennebaker J, eds. *Handbook of Mental Control,* vol 5. Englewood Cliffs, NJ: Prentice-Hall; 1993.

4. Patterson GR. *Coercive Family Process.* Eugene, Ore: Castalia; 1982.

5. McKay M, Rogers PD, McKay J. *When Anger Hurts: Quieting the Storm Within.* Oakland, Calif: New Harbinger Press; 1989.

6. Mallick SK, McCandless BR. A study of catharsis aggression. *J Pers Soc Psychol.* 1966;4:591-596.

7. Tarvis C. *Anger: The Misunderstood Emotion.* New York, NY: Simon & Schuster; 1982.

8. Williams R, Williams V. *Anger Kills.* New York, NY: Harper Perennial; 1993.

9. Matthews KA, Woodall LK. Childhood origins of overt Type A behaviors and cardiovascular reactivity to behavioral stressors. *Ann Behav Med.* 1988;10:71–77.

10. Smith TW, Anderson NB. Models of personality and disease: An interactional approach to Type A behavior and cardiovascular risk. *J Pers Soc Psychol.* 1986;3:1166–1173.

11. Tarvis C. On the wisdom of counting from one to ten. *Review Per Soc Psychol.* 1984;5:270–291.

12. Suarez E, et al. Anger increases expression of interleukin-1 on monocytes in hostile women. Paper presented at: Annual Meeting of the American Psychosomatic Society; March 1996; Williamsburg, Va.

13. Botchin MB, et al. Low versus high prolactin responders to fenfluramine challenge: Marker of behavioral differences in adult male cynomolgus macaques. *Neuropsychopharmacol.* 1993;9:93–99.

14. Smith TW. Hostility and health: Current status of a psychosomatic hypothesis. *Health Psychol.* 1992;11:139–150.

15. Sotile WM, Sotile MO. *The Medical Marriage: Sustaining Healthy Relationships for Physicians and Their Families.* Chicago, Ill: American Medical Association; 2000.

16. Novack D, Suchman A, et al. For the Working Group on Promoting Physician Personal Awareness, American Academy on Physician and Patient. Calibrating the physician: personal awareness and effective patient care. *JAMA*. 1997;278:502–509.

17. Alan R. Anger management: A systemic program to reduce unwanted anger. Presented at: Third National Conference of The Psychology of Health, Immunity and Disease, The National Institute for the Clinical Application of Behavioral Medicine; 1991; Orlando, Fla.

18. Sotile WM. *Heart Illness and Intimacy: How Caring Relationships Aid Recovery.* Baltimore, Md: Johns Hopkins University Press; 1992.

19. Siegman AW, Anderson RA, and Berger T. The angry voice: Its effects on the experience of anger and cardiovascular reactivity. *Psychosom Med*. 1991;52:631–643.

Negotiating Conflict

"Negotiating has become a fundamental skill that physicians need in order to survive and prosper."

Roger Dawson
The Physician Executive[1]

As the new millennium approached, it became clear that "The world of work we entered is not the one we live in today."[2 (p. 34)] Specifically referring to health care, consultant Roger Dawson put it succinctly:

> "What a difference a few years can make to a profession, which we now call an industry. An industry where hospital administrators have become corporate presidents, and describe patients as customers and diseases as product lines."[1 (p. 43)]

In this challenging environment, anger is a predictable by-product, and managing personal anger reactions is necessary, but not sufficient, if you want to stay stress hardy. Today's medical environment mandates that physician leaders become competent negotiators adept at resolving conflict. The concepts and skills described in this chapter can help you in two ways. First, using these tools can keep your relationships from becoming laden with conflict. Second, the strategies outlined below can help you to manage yourself and to positively influence others, even during the most difficult times of conflict.

HOW DO YOU VIEW CONFLICT?

The first step in effective negotiation is to accept and understand the nature of conflict.[3] Conflict is a process of polarization that happens when two parties lock into a "not enough to go around" mentality, move to opposite sides of the issue, and fortify their relative positions by overstating their case. Conflict escalates if these same parties ignore effective negotiation strategies and focus on defending their respective positions and trying to destroy the positions posed by their opponent. As explained by Marcus et al,[3] conflict is essentially a process of simplification: We ignore the reasons, viewpoints, and concerns of the other side. As a result, we become blind to the weaknesses of our own perspectives.

IS CONFLICT A PROBLEM OR AN OPPORTUNITY?

Learning to frame conflict positively is a key to EEM. If you see conflict only as a problem, you will begin to view the people involved as troublemakers, and your goal will be to silence or eliminate them.[3] On the other hand, you can better accept and manage conflict by using any of a number of positive frames of reference. *For example, you could decide that conflict is . . .*

- An opportunity to learn something about another party
- An opportunity to teach others something important about yourself
- A naturally occurring phenomenon
- An inevitability
- A time to constructively express your differences
- A way to further clarify your mutual goals, roles, and opportunities
- A barometer of what needs to be changed
- An opportunity for cooperative negotiation

PREPARING FOR NEGOTIATION

According to conflict consultant Rick Schroeder,[4] physicians often make a fatal error when approaching a conflict negotiation: They assume that, due to their intelligence, education, and experience, they can enter a negotiation and figure out the other party's needs, desires, objectives, motives, and interests on the spot.

In truth, effective negotiators prepare for negotiation by gathering relevant information about the other party or parties and about their desired outcome before entering into the negotiation. In complex negotiations (eg, with hospital administrators, insurance representatives, or potential employers), you might need to utilize specialized business or medical libraries, online services, inside reports, or published articles or papers regarding the topic. At minimum, conflict consultants[3,5,6] suggest that honestly answering the following questions will help you to better prepare for any conflict negotiation.

1. *Are all parties interested in resolving this productively?* If not, no negotiation strategy in the world will produce positive outcomes. Instead, negotiating a settlement might require the help of a professional mediator, arbitrator, or counselor.

2. *What does the other side want?* Beware of assuming that you know the answer to this question. Start by listing your hunches and intuitions, but remember to check these out during your dealings with the other party. Ask yourself the following:

   - What do I assume the other party most wants?
   - Is it reasonable?
   - What am I willing to give in the direction of what the other side wants?
   - How can we come up with a better deal for both of us?
   - What would work best for the other party?
   - How can we get the other party what they need?

3. *What does the other side value?* We feel a kinship with others who respect our values. On the other hand, acrimonious feelings are stirred by people who disrespect us. Remember, "The people you negotiate with will go to extraordinary lengths to help and assist you if they truly like you."[7] In this regard, effective negotiators tend to be empathic people, not simply hard-nosed debaters.

4. *What is the best possible outcome realistically available for both parties?* Frame the negotiation by looking at the problem from the future perspective, then negotiate backward. Only when you can conceptualize a win–win or a "good enough" outcome will you be able to negotiate a settlement that is acceptable to all concerned.

5. *Whose problem is this?* In most conflicts, one party is more invested in negotiating change, while the other party is more satisfied with the status quo. If you are in the latter position, resist the temptation to present a "take it or leave it" ultimatum. Doing so might win this argument, but this style of

dominating will surely damage your relationship and impede future negotiations when the roles might be reversed. Ask yourself the following:

- What elements of the situation am I able and willing to change?
- What matters most to me/to the other party in this situation?
- What is at stake for me/for the other party in this situation?

6. *What do I know about the conflict management style of the other party?* It is an adage in the counseling profession that you must match before you can lead. Unless you convey a sincere understanding of and appreciation of the other person's perspective on a given problem, you are unlikely to succeed in your efforts to shift their perspective.

From personal experience, you probably already know much about how loved ones and close associates are likely to react during conflict; you have amassed experiences that allow you to consciously or intuitively know the paradigms that shape the responses of those close acquaintances. Some are optimistic, some pessimistic; some are logical, others emotional; some are conciliatory, others argumentative. You probably use this knowledge intuitively as you deal with these people.

More difficult to predict are the response sets of strangers. Throughout history, it has been human nature to view others who differ from ourselves with suspicion and to assume that we must protect ourselves from "them." However, cross-cultural studies have shown that, regardless of the outer trappings of style, most people through all ages, from all walks of life, and from various cultures are more similar than different from each other. Specifically, we want to be understood, to attain safety, to protect our loved ones and our personal interests, and to be respected.[8]

This notion of similarity of underlying interests notwithstanding, it also appears that, as groups, certain professions within health care tend to assume predictable "postures" when engaged in conflict. These conflict postures may be the cumulative result of educational experiences, personality characteristics, or implicit or explicit social mores operative in different professions and work milieus. Regardless of their cause, and despite the fact that

TABLE 8-1

Characteristic Tendencies

Physicians	Administrators/Managers	Nurses
Doers	Planners	Processors
Work in a one-on-one relationship	Work as a director of a group	Work in collaboration with others
Reactive	Proactive	Reactive
Immediate gratification	Delayed gratification	Immediate gratification
Deciders	Delegators	Implementors
Independent	Participative	Collaborative
Problem solving/solo	Problem solving/team	Problem solving/team
Business owners	Business stewards	Employees
Value collegiality	Value collaboration	Value professional validation

Source: Wong BD. Collegiality and collaboration. Handout from a Workshop presentation to Medical Group Management Association Regional Meeting; 1999; Dallas, TX. Used with permission.

many exceptions to these stereotypes exist, we still propose that it is helpful for physicians to respect certain tendencies. Table 8-1 represents our modification of a similar list regarding physicians and administrators offered by Brian D. Wong, Partner and National Director, Physician Services, Arthur Andersen LLP.[9]

Our consulting experiences suggest that the most profound shift in interpersonal dynamics that has occurred in health care during the past two decades involves physician–nurse relationships. Stein and colleagues[10,11] noted that, in the late 1960s, the nurse was not allowed to have an independent opinion regarding treatment of the patient. The traditional, rigid hierarchy that heretofore defined physician–nurse relationships promoted what the authors described as "a transactional neurosis" in which nurses could make only concealed suggestions. Now, nurses are assertively claiming their professional turf as valued collaborators in the delivery of whole-person care to medical patients. This fact, coupled with our ongoing shortage of nurses—a situation that is predicted to continue into the indefinite future—requires new skills for promoting collegiality between the two professions.

There is no place in the contemporary physician–nurse relationship for a closed, nonaffirming interpersonal style. O'Mara[12] cautioned that authoritarian attitudes by physicians put any medical institution at risk for low nursing staff morale. Rather, efforts should be made to involve nurses in collaborative interdisciplinary care plans.

THE IMPORTANCE OF REHEARSAL

How many complex skills have you mastered without practicing them? As with learning anything new, it is important to rehearse how you plan to behave during a tough negotiation. Practice how you plan to respond to specific, upcoming situations with patients, loved ones, or adversaries. Role play your reactions. Picture yourself responding in ways that are effective. For example, you might use these techniques to prepare for a scheduled follow-up to deal with a specific conflict:

- Set aside a 15- to 30-minute block of time to quietly prepare for the encounter.
- List what points you want to get across in the follow-up.
- Recall what you know about effective versus ineffective ways of dealing with conflict.

Specify how you would like to behave as you are conveying these points. Then practice behaving in these ways.

- Some of this practice should be behavioral. Stand before a mirror and pretend that you are dealing with the person with whom you have scheduled the follow-up. As you rehearse, notice yourself from the perspectives outlined in Table 7-1.
- Next, relax and use mental imagery to see, hear, and feel yourself dealing effectively in this situation. Replay a positive mental image until you can comfortably imagine yourself dealing effectively with the situation.

Practicing in this way has an added benefit. Soon the skills that you develop while rehearsing for anticipated situations become habits that serve you well in the heat of unanticipated bouts of anger.

NEGOTIATING CONFLICT WITHOUT DAMAGING RELATIONSHIPS

In transient relationships, disagreements are often ignored or dismissed. We wisely reason that it simply is not worth the effort it takes to deal with every disagreement that comes our way. But in an ongoing personal or professional relationship, if you ignore, dismiss, or demean, you run the risk of turning a momentary "bump" in rapport into festering conflict. The seven guidelines for cooperative negotiation discussed following can help you to resolve differences without hurting your relationships.[5,13,14]

Guideline 1: Practice Being an Effective Emotional Manager

Even a minor irritant can trigger a full-blown anger reaction when you are already overstressed. On the other hand, you are more likely to deal effectively with even the most challenging conflict if you are in reasonable emotional control to start with. Important, too, is to be honest about your own interpersonal style.

Schroeder[4] underscored the importance of resisting the temptation to assume a role in negotiation that is not natural for your personality. Doing so will not only stress you, it will also diminish your effectiveness as a negotiator.

Guideline 2: Respect Your Physiology

If you tend to have exaggerated fight-or-flight reactions and impoverished calming reactions, it is especially important not to stoke your fires of anger. As you prepare for a difficult meeting, beware of stimulants like caffeine, nicotine, and simple sugars. These can magnify an already-existing supercharged nervous system. Also, remember that doing and thinking more than one thing at once activates a stress response. Prepare for your meeting by taking a break to clear your mind. If possible, make time to wash stress out of your body with exercise or relaxation.

Guideline 3: Learn to Detach

You will be better able to maintain control and negotiate effectively if you can detach yourself from the situation or person that is making you angry. As a physician, you are probably already quite proficient in using this coping tool. "Therapeutic detachment" is a survival skill used when performing medical procedures. Remember to use this same skill during negotiations.

Ury[15] suggests that you "go to the balcony" and get a view of the conflict from a distance, especially noting how the dispute looks from that vantage point and the experience of the other party. Alternatively, in your mind's eye, you might pretend that you are watching a movie of you and the person with whom you are interacting.[16] Pretend that you are in the audience, calmly watching the two of you up on the screen. This allows you to experience the interaction from a one-step-removed position—a position in which it is much easier to control your emotions. Be honest as you evaluate how your behavior may contribute to the dynamics of the conflict. Do you convey a respect of the people involved in the conflict? Does your negotiating style leave a way for the other party to save face, regardless of the outcome of the negotiation?

Guideline 4: Listen to Yourself

While you are depersonalizing the situation with imagery, control your self-talk. Use the anger-managing coping statements listed in Chapter 7.

Guideline 5: Strike While the Iron Is Warm

Truly powerful and assertive people choose their times for dealing with conflict. Use your own good judgment as to when you will be at your best to negotiate a complex issue. Ideally, stewing disagreements should be nipped in the bud, before they fester into full-blown conflicts. And once conflict does occur, it is crucial *not* to strike while the iron is hot. Consider the following formula for responding: Call time-out before responding; schedule a time to follow-up with the person; then collect your thoughts and your emotions and wait until your anger calms before engaging the other party in negotiation.

   We emphasize that it is okay to show emotion during negotiations, but you mustn't lose control to the point that you say or do something that you might later regret. Remember: "A second of patience when you're angry will save you 100 days of sorrow" (Chinese proverb).

Guideline 6: Deal with One Issue at a Time

Resist the temptation to let conflict about one issue lead into a shower of attacks and counterattacks about multiple concerns. As tensions escalate, we all tend to throw unfinished business into the current conversation. Looking backward during an argument only serves to escalate defensiveness and conflict. Look forward. Talk about what you would like to see happen relevant to the current issue under discussion, not about past resentments. Don't try to resolve everything during one negotiation; doing so only muddies the water and makes it difficult to resolve anything.

Remember that every important issue deserves its own discussion. If a new issue surfaces during negotiations or if your discussion calls up pain you have been harboring from a past dealing with this person, that topic deserves a separate discussion. Flag it and make either a mental note or a contract with the other party to return to this point in the near future.

> Example: "That raises an important related point that I'd like to pursue in a future discussion. I need to sleep on that one. Could we meet again tomorrow to specifically address that issue? For now, I'd like for us to stay focused on the topic at hand."

Guideline 7: Separate the Person From the Problem

In their helpful book *Getting to Yes*, authors Roger Fisher and William Ury[17] emphasize that effective negotiating starts by separating the person from the problem. This involves working to create an "us versus the problem" attitude and avoiding a "me versus you" mentality. You can do this by using these six simple communication strategies:

1. *Stroke the person and show a leap of faith that you will resolve the problem at hand.*

   > Example: "I know that you're doing what you think is best. I never question your integrity or the fact that you will do whatever you believe will be helpful. I trust that we will be able to resolve this, even though we disagree about what would be the most helpful thing to do. This really is bothering me, though, and I appreciate your willingness to work through this with me."

2. *Listen.* Listening allows you to gather important information that is missed if you are constantly talking or stuck in your own racing thoughts, preparing your counter for as soon as the other person's lips stop moving. Be quiet, and *listen!* This is such a difficult and important interpersonal skill that we

have devoted an entire chapter to the topic. For now, two thoughts on the matter of listening: "Silence is a potent strategic weapon. . .Just as nature abhors a vacuum, a weak negotiator abhors silence. . .Above all, you need to avoid the temptation to prove how smart [or tough] you are by continuously talking."[7] More to the point: "Listen or your tongue will make you go deaf."(Manatova Chief)

3. *Validate the other person's perceptions.* If the other person is convinced that you truly understand and have empathy for their point of view, their defensiveness will lower and they will be more open to understanding *your* point of view. Use words that convey respect, empathy, and compassion for the other person's point.

   Example: "When I put myself in your shoes, I can understand why you must think or feel what you do. Your points are well made and well received. I see things somewhat differently, but I can understand your perspective, too."

4. *Don't blame or shame.* In our experience, physicians who were subjected to excessive criticism in their professional or personal formation tend to approach conflict with a mentality of "Find out whose to blame, and blame that sucker!" The quest to assign culpability obscures the true point of negotiation: resolving an issue without damaging relationships. Help the other party to save face as you negotiate. This is an effective way to build mutual respect and trust, assets that will serve you well when the need for future conflict resolution arises.

   Example: "Regardless of how we got here, it is important to me that we resolve this. I assume that you feel the same way. I'm invested in working with you to figure out a way to resolve this that leaves you knowing that I respect you and that leaves me feeling that you hold me in a similar regard."

5. *Emphasize where you agree.* Negotiation will go more smoothly if you and the other party stand on common ground as you attempt to resolve your differences. It's a mistake to emphasize where you *disagree* before underscoring where you *agree.*

   Example: "I know that we have our differences about this matter, but let's not lose sight of the fact that, in truth, we agree more than we disagree. We seem to agree that (a) this is a problem that we need to solve together, (b) we care enough about our relationship to want to resolve this, and (c) we share the opinion(s) that (fill in the blank) might be helpful."

6. *Apologize.* This is not the same as admitting fault or letting the other party off the hook. Apologizing simply involves stating that you are sorry you are having this conflict. Doing so is a very powerful way to calm otherwise disturbed waters in any relationship. Remember: The most powerful words in any language are "I'm sorry."

Example: "I'm sorry that we're going through this right now. I know that neither of us likes it when we argue." Or: "I'm really sorry that we're having this problem with (fill in the blank). It's not very pleasant for either of us to have to deal with this."

Guideline 8: Clarify Underlying Issues

Fisher and Ury pointed out the dangers of negotiating from "postures" rather than taking the time and effort to identify your own and the other party's underlying issues. In a nutshell, effective negotiation requires that you not get stuck in an angry posture that simply fuels further anger. Try to identify and communicate about your own and the other person's underlying needs during conflict. In noninflammatory language, clarify your position and reflect an awareness of the other person's position.

CLOSING ACTS

The final stages of negotiation are crucial to ensuring that the discussion enhances, rather than harms, your relationship. In formal negotiations, it is always wise to take notes and turn them into a memorandum that outlines your understanding of what was negotiated. Doing so creates a mechanism for clarifying any differences in interpretation and creates documentation that might serve you well during future negotiations. In less formal situations, it is always wise to follow up a conflict discussion with a note, phone call, or face-to-face encounter during which you express appreciation for having had the discussion and ask how the other person is feeling about the issues you discussed. Do this soon after the conflict. The longer you wait, the more awkward you are likely to feel in future dealings with the other person.

Finally, remember that dealing with conflict is not an event; it is a process that requires follow-up. When done appropriately, conflict negotiation can actually strengthen your relationship with the other party. Trust, respect, and appreciation of each other's

T A B L E   8-2

Do's and Don'ts for Effective Anger Management and Conflict Negotiation

Do:

Listen

Stay calm

Choose your time to respond

Emphasize where you agree

Stroke the other person

Separate person from problem

Establish norms that are positive regarding behavioral expectations of self and others "We expect. . ."

Respect confidentiality

Give feedback regularly

Stay focused on one issue at a time

Limit the number of issues addressed in one session

Build a storehouse of positives in the relationship

Communicate regularly

Identify your own and other's underlying issues

Stay curious about opinions and perceptions that differ from your own

Don't:

Coerce and bully

Criticize

Cut off

Strike while the iron is hot

Hang onto hurt

Live in toxic relationships

Discount (underestimate) the other side

Interrupt

Lock into a "position"

Exaggerate

Blame

Make excuses

Restrict the flow of information

Restrict participation in important decisions

Create us-versus-them distinctions

Discredit others

Undermine and sabotage others

Express cynicism

Be indirect in your communication style

Show no positive response to input or suggestions

Give inconsistent or mixed messages

integrity come with resolution of conflict. Follow up to ensure that the agreements made during negotiations were implemented, to express appreciation for your last meeting, and to check whether further issues remain to be resolved. Meet regularly to ensure that problems do not fester. Negotiating is easiest when it begins early in the lifecycle of a conflict.

CONCLUSIONS

The self-assessment and negotiation strategies outlined in this chapter and the two preceding chapters can help you to move beyond struggling with episodes of conflict to shaping truly stress-resilient relationships. See Table 8-2 for a reminder list of Do's and Don'ts.[3,6,18]

REFERENCES—CHAPTER 8

1. Dawson R, Why do physicians have difficulty negotiating? *The Physician Executive.* 1999;25:43–44.
2. Reinhold BB. *Toxic Work.* New York, NY: Dutton; 1996.
3. Marcus L, Dorn BC, Kritek PB, Miller VG, Wyatt JB. *Renegotiating Health Care: Resolving Conflict to Build Collaboration.* San Francisco, Calif: Jossey-Bass; 1995.
4. Schroeder RE. *Communicate and Negotiate.* Englewood, Colo: Medical Group Management Association; 1999.
5. Linney BJ. The successful physician negotiator. *The Physician Executive.* 1999;25:62–65.
6. Aschenbrener CA, Siders CT. Managing low-to-mid intensity conflict in the health care setting. *The Physician Executive.* 1999;25:44–50.
7. Babitsky S, Mangraviti JJ. *The Successful Physician Negotiator: How to Get What You Deserve.* Falmouth, Mass: SEAK, Inc; 1998.
8. Csikszentmihalyi M. *Finding Flow.* New York, NY: Basic Books; 1997.
9. Wong BD. Collegiality and collaboration. Workshop presentation to Medical Group Management Association Regional Meeting; 1999; Dallas, Texas.
10. Stein L. The doctor-nurse game. *Arch Gen Psychiatry.* 1967;16:699.
11. Stein L, Watts D, Howell T. The doctor-nurse game revisited. *N Engl J Med.* 1990;322:546.
12. O'Mara K. Communication and conflict resolution in emergency medicine. *Emerg Med Clin North Am.* 1999;17:451–459.
13. Sotile WM, Sotile MO. The angry physician: I. The temper-tantruming physician. *The Physician Executive.* 1996;22:30–34.
14. Sotile WM, Sotile MO. The angry physician: II. Managing yourself while managing others. *The Physician Executive.* 1996;22:39–42.
15. Ury W. *Getting Past No: Negotiating with Difficult People.* New York, NY: Bantam Books; 1991.
16. Grinder J, Bandler R. *Trance-Formations: Neuro-Linguistic Programming and the Structure of Hypnosis.* Moab, Utah: Real People Press; 1981.
17. Fisher R, Ury W. *Getting to Yes,* 2nd ed. New York, NY: Penguin Books; 1991.
18. Ryan KD, Oestreich DK. *Driving Fear Out of the Workplace,* 2nd ed. San Francisco, Calif: Jossey-Bass; 1998.

chapter | 9

The Disruptive Physician

"The age of the cowboy surgeon is over."

Wayne and Mary Sotile

Yesterday's freewheeling, independent, straight-talking physician runs the risk today of being labeled a disruptive physician. The mandate for increased collaboration and cross-disciplinary respectfulness in the medical workplace constitutes a call to physicians to better manage their own and each other's behaviors. Doing so can prove to be a formidable task.

In hopes of easing this process, we offer suggestions for ways to recognize, understand, and intervene to prevent or curb disruptive physician behaviors. Before defining our terms, we offer the reminder that the vast majority of physicians are caring, courteous professionals. No definitive statistics are available regarding the incidence of disruptive physician behavior, but it is generally thought that fewer than 10% of physicians evidence disruptive behavior.[1] But the disruption to collegiality and collaboration that results from this powerful few can seriously erode the resilience of any medical organization.

WHAT IS DISRUPTIVE PHYSICIAN BEHAVIOR?

Springer and Casale[2] offered the following legalistic description of the disruptive physician:

> "The disruptive practitioner is by definition contentious, threatening, unreachable, insulting, and frequently litigious. He will not, or cannot, play by the rules, nor is he able to relate to or work well with others. . ... It is not uncommon to find that a disruptive practitioner is, in fact, highly intelligent, clinically superior, even medically outstanding. However...his inability to get along with others sometimes affects his clinical judgment. He is totally convinced that he is right. Those who would question him or seek to have him behave differently, whether they

are colleagues or not, are seen to be motivated by ignorance, stupidity, jealousy, or a desire to destroy him as an economic competitor. They are also believed to be weak and vulnerable. He may not openly take on the strong and prestigious, but rather seek to undermine and intimidate those who can neither avoid him nor fight back...."

Springer and Casale go on to caution that a libelous situation develops if the disrupter's personal idiosyncrasies begin to affect the ability of others to get their jobs done or when such idiosyncrasies begin to interfere with the practitioner's ability to perform well professionally.

In their worst moments, disrupters deal with interpersonal tensions by bullying. They create fear and seek obedience with an intimidating or abusive management style. At other times, a disrupter's grossly offensive language, habits, demeanor, or behavior leads to discomfort for those around them. In one way or another, a disrupter's demoralizing tactics keep relationships embroiled in conflict, simmering with tension, or steaming in the aftereffects of yet another outburst.

We emphasize that disruptive behavior is not limited to blatant acts of aggression or verbal abuse. Physicians can also be labeled disruptive for behaviors like the following:[3]

- Excessively flirting
- Being sexually suggestive or assaultive
- Recurring dishonesty and projection of blame for failure
- Racial, cultural, or sexual bias that precludes development of a team relationship with fellow professionals and/or affects evenness of clinical care across patient populations
- Unreliability or inability to lead a health care team
- Refusing to see certain categories of patients
- Making disparaging comments about colleagues or hospital personnel or administrators
- Not responding to input or suggestions from partners
- Acting cold, aloof
- Being passive–aggressive, eg, chronic absence or tardiness from group meetings or refusal to participate in organizational team-building efforts
- Refusing to follow group policies

TABLE 9-1

Characteristics of Disrupters

Instructions: Check any of the following statements that apply to the person being evaluated.

___ Regularly creates situations that lead to patient dissatisfaction, staff and colleagues reaching their wits' end, and/or administrators feeling paralyzed.

___ Habitually denies to self and others the wrongful nature of his or her actions and externalizes responsibility for those behaviors.

___ Repeatedly justifies disruptive behavior by blaming co-workers, administrators, working conditions, patients, or other events.

___ Responds to reasonable efforts by others to confront his or her inappropriate behavior by setting up covert threats of retaliation or even self-harm.

___ Overtly uses his or her professional status or powerful personality to silence criticism.

___ Resists any monitoring of his or her behavior by challenging the authority of those who order it and finds loopholes in the behavioral requirements.

___ Is hypersensitive to criticism. As a result, any intervention attempt heightens shameful feelings that fuel even more problematic behavior.

Source: Gendel MH. Disruptive behaviors, personality problems, and boundary violations. In: Goldman L, Myers M, Dickstein L, eds. *The Handbook of Physician Health.* Chicago, Ill: American Medical Association; 2000:138–160.

Use the checklist in Table 9-1 to assess yourself or a colleague regarding the disruptive behavior syndrome.

HOW DANGEROUS IS DISRUPTIVE BEHAVIOR?

At minimum, disruptive behavior creates workplace stress that can diminish morale, productivity, and quality of care in any medical setting. At its worse, disruptive behavior creates vulnerability to disciplinary action from one's organization or legal action. "There is now a substantial body of case law that emphasizes that disruptive behavior is sufficient to warrant a physicians exclusion from the medical staff."[2]

Consultants caution that legally actionable, disruptive behaviors in the workplace must be differentiated from those that are simply unpleasant or obnoxious. Behaviors that are considered "actionable" by legal experts[5,6] are outlined below:

- Personal and unprofessional verbal attacks
- Impertinent and inappropriate comments written in medical records

- Sexual harassment of medical/hospital staff or patients
- Intimidating, belittling, nonconstructive criticism
- Requiring unnecessarily burdensome activities of staff that have nothing to do with patient care
- Public criticism of other physicians, hospitals, or personnel that occurs outside of appropriate channels
- Refusal to accept medical staff assignments or doing so in a disruptive manner

WHAT CAUSES DISRUPTIVE BEHAVIORS?

Most physicians are caring people. Even disrupters tend to be attempting to show that they care about protecting their turf, about their patient's safety, or about the quality of their profession. The problem is that they express their concerns in ways that complicate relationships rather than solve problems. It is also true that anyone who evidences repeated bouts of disruptive behavior may be battling complicated internal and/or organizational "demons."

Physician Kent Neff, an expert in assessing disruptive physicians, asserts that chronically disruptive behaviors are often linked to developmental roots, including a history of having been abused or deprived. This may result in a limited capacity for empathy and a relatively low "emotional IQ." Because they simply don't see how their behavior affects others, chronic disrupters, even during the best of times, tend to have difficulty dealing effectively with relationships. Neff claims that most of the disruptive physicians he has evaluated evidenced excessive work coupled with low self-esteem and a general sense of ineffectiveness and powerlessness that contributed to states of depression and substance abuse.[7]

Unfortunately, their boorish behavior often obscures the fact that, due to their lack of adequate coping skills, disruptive physicians often suffer great stress and personal pain. Five "demons" that may fuel disruptive behavior are: mismanaged stress, substance abuse, character disorders and trait anger, marital–family tensions, and immaturity.[7]

Mismanaged Stress

In our opinion, outbursts of disruptive behavior are at least triggered by, if not wholly caused by, excessive or poorly managed
stress. We assume that by now it is clear that we believe that the
work demands and corresponding emotional wear and tear experienced by most physicians are extraordinary and generally
underestimated. Many disruptive physicians we counsel bring to
mind notions of soldiers who have spent far too long "on point"
in a war: They've acclimated to a state of chronic stress arousal
that predisposes them to "shoot the first thing that moves."

Substance Abuse

Nearly 75% of physicians who come before their state medical
boards for behavioral problems are there because of problems
involving the abuse of alcohol or other drugs.[8] However, it is
often difficult to discern when this is the case. It is relatively easy
to detect an actively intoxicated physician. But what about a
physician who often shows up at work irritable, demanding, and
defensive? Is such a person's foul mood due to a hangover? Or is
this simply another exhausted, stressed physician doing his or her
best to make it through another day? This differentiation needs to
be considered with care.

Character Disorders and Trait Anger

Character-disordered people basically fail to learn from experience. When faced with negative outcomes, their narcissistic
worldview leads to excessive justification of inappropriate,
exploitive behavior and projection of blame onto others.

   High trait anger, or the tendency to experience anger across
situations, can occur both independently and in conjunction with
character disorder pathology. As was mentioned in our discussion
of stress resilience (Chapter 4), individuals who score high on measures of trait anger have been shown to engage in more counterproductive work behavior, such as arguing with others or sabotaging
their work, than those who are not elevated on trait anger. In addition, high trait anger has been found to correlate strongly with
aggressive acts against both the organization and other people.[9]

Marital–Family Tensions

Recent research has suggested a link between workplace violence and marital-family dysfunction. Brown[10] analyzed nearly 1,000 cases of enacted or threatened workplace violence recorded in human resource records of a number of Fortune 500 companies. Remarkably, he found that in only 6% of cases were job issues identified as the primary cause for threats or acts of violence. But in fully 74% of threatened or enacted workplace violence cases, domestic disputes had occurred the night before the incident. Brown concluded that it appears that many disrupters enter the workplace with the attitude "I might have to put up with all of this grief at home, but I'll be damned if I'll tolerate anything from you people at work."

One physician who had recently separated from his wife after a lengthy dysfunctional marriage disclosed to us that

"without question, the majority of those disruptive incident reports filed against me in the hospital had to do with my displaced anger. I remember so many times when I left home infuriated with my wife. As I headed out to the hospital, instead of dealing honestly with my grief and frustration about my home life, I'd let myself work up anger about work. Many times, by the time I got to the hospital, I had concocted intricate scenarios in my head of what might happen at work that would infuriate me. I'd hit the hospital doors loaded with anger. Then I'd look for some place to discharge my rage."

Immaturity

To a large extent, psychosocial and psychosexual maturity comes from accumulated interpersonal experiences across a variety of contexts. The fact that medical training is extraordinarily time-consuming and demanding and that it typically persists until one's early 30s, leaves many physicians with a limited range of role-related skills and a relatively low level of maturity when they enter medical practice.[11] One perspective on disruptive behavior is that it is essentially an immature reaction to interpersonal stress.

In this regard, anecdotal experiences with chronically disruptive physicians sometimes has called to mind the findings from research with aggressive high-school students. Slaby and Guerra[12] reported that high-school "bullies" tend to have a common mind-set: When they encounter interpersonal tensions, they immediately jump to conclusions about the other person's hostility

TABLE 9-2

Old and New Paradigms for Understanding Physician Behavior

Old Paradigm	New Paradigm
This physician is just a "jerk."	This physician needs help.
This problem is hopeless.	This problem is possibly an opportunity.
Disruptive physicians are bad physicians.	Most often, these are good physicians.
We need new data before acting.	An incident should lead to examining all data already existent regarding this physician's behavior.
Exercise extreme caution before intervening.	Implement fast, firm action.
Let's manage this one event.	Manage the processes that led to, and that may result from, this event.

Source: Neff KE, Samoulis S, Widra L. Managing disruptive behavior in the hospital. Presented to: VHA Leadership Conference; April 16–19, 2000; Dallas, TX. Used with permission.

toward them. They do not consider alternative explanations for the other person's behavior that might lead to peaceful settlement of their differences. Further, they deny the negative consequences of acting out their anger. Instead, they justify their aggressive behavior with self-statements such as "It's better to fight it out than to lose face" or "The consequences of the fight can't be that bad."

Our consulting experiences suggest another important point about disruptive physicians whose behavior may be due to relative immaturity: They are generally unhappy with their lack of self-control and are receptive to learning better coping strategies.

A NEW PARADIGM FOR UNDERSTANDING DISRUPTIVE PHYSICIANS

Neff et al[7] recommended a new paradigm for understanding disruptive physician behavior. The contrasts between the old and new paradigms are outlined in Table 9-2.

We add to this schemata an expansion of the traditional notion that disruptive behavior is the problem of an individual. We propose instead that it is both more realistic and helpful to view disruptive behavior as the tip of an iceberg, the understructure of which is some combination of psychological, family, and perhaps organizational factors. Accordingly, prevention and remediation of disruptive workplace behavior requires a combined approach. Confronting the disruptive physician with limit-setting interventions is necessary. But disrupters must also be helped to build more adaptive coping skills and to address the issues that underlie their problem behaviors. In addition, if various physicians in your organization evidence disruptive behavior, it calls into question the healthiness of your organization. In this situation, it is wise to consider whether the disruptive behavior is a symptom of a system's problem, not just a cause of problems within the system. It is both unfair and unrealistic to expect an individual to learn to function adaptively in an unhealthy environment. Unless your organizational culture promotes positive interpersonal dynamics, you will be doomed to a series of episodes of conflict, each an indicator of an unhealthy workplace.

Finally, every medical organization must assure its members adequate protection from disruptive individuals. Guidelines for providing such protection follow.

PROTECTING YOUR ORGANIZATION

Seventy percent of workers in corporate America fear that if they speak up and complain about how they are being treated, they will suffer retaliation.[3] A clearly stated code of conduct and policies and procedures for dealing with its violation are necessary if employees are to be freed of this fear. In prior writings,[13,14] we offered the following recommendations for how to do just that.

Writing a Code of Conduct

The notion of a code of conduct stirs waves of opposition from most physicians. No medical group wants to be ruled by overbearing, intrusive monitoring procedures.

It is important to see an organizational code of conduct as a mechanism of protection, not constraint. It is also important to be proactive. If you wait to adopt a code of conduct in the wake of a complaint, the offending party is likely to perceive the policy as being a punitive, personal attack.[15,16]

In general, the code should flow logically from your organization's mission statement. It should specify what is expected of each member of your work team. It is advisable to call attention

F I G U R E   9-1

Sample Mission Statement and Code of Conduct

Mission Statement

The mission of Practice X is to provide the highest quality of medical care that is consistently delivered with courtesy, professionalism, and positive collaboration with our medical community.

In addition, we commit to promoting and protecting the positive reputation and operation of our organization.

Policy Statement

To satisfy our mission, employees of Practice X must treat patients, staff, and fellow physicians in a dignified manner that conveys respect for the abilities of each other and a willingness to work together as a team. Behavior that is deemed to be disruptive to promoting an atmosphere of collegiality, cooperation, and professionalism will not be tolerated. It is expected that employees of Practice X will devote the time and resources necessary to achieve these goals.

to both blatantly unacceptable behaviors—like impairment from substance abuse or sexual harassment—and those behaviors that can subtly damage your organization's morale, productivity, or reputation.[3] Typically, such codes are brief and to the point. Figure 9-1 is a sample mission statement with an accompanying code of conduct.

Guidelines for Developing Policies and Procedures

Keep three things in mind as you develop or implement procedures for reporting inappropriate behavior:

1. Make it easy, and confidential. Your complaint system should be uncomplicated and should protect a complainant's privacy.[17] And remember that unless staff members and physicians are trained in how to use the reporting process, it is useless.
2. Assure prompt and regular feedback. Both the complainant and the target of the complaint need to know what is being done in response to the charge. At minimum, give the physician prompt feedback that a complaint has been filed, interview him or her

regarding the incident, and indicate if and when further inquiries or meetings will be held. Also update the complainant, even if all that can be said is simply, "We are not ignoring your complaint. I'm sorry that I can't say more at this time. But please know that we are following through; we have taken your complaint seriously."

3. You may need the help of a special committee. Forming a special committee charged specifically with the task of overseeing interpersonal relations may be helpful. In hospitals, this committee is typically comprised of representatives from the boards of key medical groups, the hospital's physician executive, a person from human resources, and an attorney. Within a medical group practice, this committee typically consists of elected physician representatives, the organizations chief administrator, and, often, an outside consultant who has expertise in behavioral management issues. We offer guidelines for the structure and operation of this committee in Chapter 13.

Pfifferling[16] offered helpful guidelines for developing a policy for managing disruptive workplace behavior. The following questions can guide you in your efforts to create an equitable system for dealing with disruptive colleagues:

1. What pattern or single incident of transgression will warrant confrontation?
2. Is an annual performance appraisal the appropriate time to confront the disruptive physician or do certain transgressions or complaints warrant immediate confrontation?
3. Who will initially contact the disruptive physician?
4. What steps will be included in the grievance process?
5. Will mediation be offered?
6. What types of options will be made available to the disruptive physician to correct his or her deficiencies?
7. At what point should the disruptive physician be sent to an outside source for assessment and assistance? How will this outside source be chosen? Should this assessment include a full complement of diagnostic tests? Who will pay for these services?

8. If the disruptive physician does not cooperate, what are the bottom lines for the practice and the individual?
9. Should a behavioral contract be developed? Who will be responsible for monitoring the terms of this contract?
10. If an absence from work is warranted, what steps will be taken to facilitate the physician's re-entry?

As explained by Pfifferling,

"Answers to these and similar questions will help...ensure that the policy addresses such key areas as behavioral expectations, method of confrontation, grievance process, assessment, treatment, sanctions, and work re-entry."[16 (p. 90)]

HOW TO RESPOND TO A COMPLAINT ABOUT DISRUPTIVE BEHAVIOR

Resist the temptation to placate, ignore, patronize, or discount someone who complains to you about a colleague's disruptive behavior. Never try to smooth the complainant's ruffled feathers with statements like, "Now you know that Dr X doesn't mean to be that way. He (or she) just tends to blow off steam like that." No matter how well intended, such responses can be construed as tacit endorsement of the inappropriate behavior and leave the complainant unsupported and you liable for contributing to a hostile work environment.

On the other hand, it is prudent to assume that your colleagues are innocent unless they are proven guilty of disruptive behavior. Do not overtly or, by implication, condemn a physician colleague. Remember that people in conflict tend to prefer to complain to a third party, rather than dealing directly with each other. Resist the pull to participate in conflict-escalating communication triangles When dealing with complainants, we recommend that you listen, empathize, and assure that appropriate action will be taken.[14] Consider the following approaches:

■ Stay calm while the complainant expresses his or her concern and listen actively. Reflect what you hear and show empathy for the speaker.
■ Express regret that this conflict has happened, but do not use inflammatory words and do not assume a collusive posture. Try to maintain the stance of someone who will facilitate

resolution of the conflict, not that of a rescuer or persecutor of any party.

- Ask what the person would like for you to do to resolve the problem. Stay focused on the specific problem at hand and state your intention to do all that you can to facilitate resolution.
- Only commit to doing what is doable.
- Emphasize your belief that, with the help of the administrative structure your organization has in place, this issue can be resolved and all parties concerned will learn something positive from this experience.

GUIDELINES FOR INTERVENING WITH A DISRUPTIVE COLLEAGUE

Avoid three fundamental mistakes when confronting disruptive colleagues. First, don't wait too long before confronting the disrupter. Remember: It is more effective to strike while the iron is warm—before tensions reach a boiling point.

Second, never blame or shame. Disruptive behavior is intolerable in today's medical workplace. However, retaliatory, vindictive, or punitive responses to offensive behavior may serve a policing function, but they do not foster the development of a positive interpersonal culture. Once again, physician leaders can learn a lesson from research in corporate America. Inept criticisms were given as the number one cause of conflict on the job by 108 managers and white-collar workers, above mistrust, personality struggles, disputes over power, and disputes over pay.[18] Clearly, *how* you offer criticism is just as important as setting limits on inappropriate behavior.

Finally, we remind you to avoid the use of vague terminology when confronting a colleague. It is possible to be sensitive, yet firm, and specific in your confrontation. Vague, tentative, or indirect confrontations seldom work, especially with an individual who is defensive or denying.

Following is advice from various experts[3,7,13-17,19,20] about how to intervene with a disruptive colleague.

Determine Who to Include in the Confrontation

Don't do it alone. A group confrontation provides more balance and force, and group input is harder to deny or dismiss as being a

personal disagreement. Include a supporter of the person to be
confronted, but be sure the supporter does not condone or minimize the bad behavior. Try not to make the meeting too con-
tentious. Keep out the offender's lawyers, at least at first.

Determine How to Orchestrate the Confrontation

Thank the physician for attending the meeting. Offer the assur-
ance that there will be ample time in this meeting to hear all sides
of the story, but ask the physician to hear you out first.

Start by communicating the physician's value and worth to
your organization. Assure the physician of your respect for him
or her, both as a professional and as a person. Point out the
offender's special skills and characteristics and his or her particular importance to your overall operation.

Next, state your concerns about the physician's behavior.
Here, it is wise to let peers take the lead. Physicians are more
-likely to accept criticism from other physicians, nurses from
other nurses, administrators from other administrators, and so on.
With a "barrage" of feedback, have each participant cite detailed
examples of how the offender's behavior has been unacceptable
or damaging to the organization. Focus feedback on specific
behaviors that have been documented, not on personality. Do not
impugn motives; assume that the physician has good intentions.
Avoid the use of any judgmental or interrogative tones. Give
several examples of problem behaviors if possible. Deal with the
problem behaviors; do not make diagnoses. Label behavior as
"unacceptable" and explain why. Remind the offender that your
feedback is based on the norms that he/she helped develop or
agreed to upon joining your organization (ie, the code of conduct).

Take Time to Listen

Solicit the offender's side of the story. Here, you might say something like:

> "Regardless of why it happened, these inappropriate behaviors must stop now.
> However, our goal is to improve relationships in this workplace, not simply to
> police bad behavior. For this reason, we want to explore why this has happened."

Do not tolerate abusive behavior during the meeting. If the physician gets out of control, end the meeting with the statement that

another meeting will be rescheduled in the near future, at which time you expect the physician to maintain control.

Work together to create a plan for change. Here, useful questions might include:

"What do you think will happen if this does not change?"
"Have you ever faced situations like this or received this sort of feedback before? If so, what helped you to modify your behavior in the past?"
"What would help you now?"
"What new skills, support, or changes would help you?"
"What kind of support do you need from me (or us)?"

Offer Concrete Advice for Positive Change

Express confidence that the offender can and will change and offer concrete suggestions for making the desired changes. If appropriate, share from your own past experiences with same or similar situations.

Depending on the severity and duration of the problem pattern, suggest or mandate that the offender receive outside help to learn appropriate behavioral control. Make a list of mental health professionals or treatment facilities that your organization has identified as being user-friendly to physicians readily available. Resources for assessing and treating impaired physicians can be identified by contacting your state or county medical society.

Specify What Needs to Be Done for the Physician to "Clear the Record"

An intervention should not leave a disruptive physician feeling or believing that he or she has been given a life sentence. In addition to specifying what will happen if the physician continues to show disruptive behavior (eg, loss of practice privileges or termination of employment), specify (1) what steps the physician must take to demonstrate cooperation with your intervention and (2) when the physician can expect to be "off probation."

In this latter regard, many organizations specify that an episode of intervention will cease when the physician has accumulated 12 months of incident-free behavior and has adhered to any other guidelines mandated by the intervention (eg, sought counseling and granted the counselor the right to report to the organization's governing agency regarding the physician's progress).

Facilitate Face-to-Face Dealings Between the Parties in Conflict

Relationships mature if conflicting parties are helped to deal directly with each other in positive ways. Whenever possible and appropriate, facilitate face-to-face encounters. Wait to conduct this meeting until defensiveness, embarrassment, and anger have calmed.

Close with Compassion and Firmness

Close with compassion, but firmly underscore that the disruptive behavior must change. Express regret that this difficulty has occurred, and acknowledge that the offender is a good person who has made poor choices. Challenge the offender to shape up or else face progressively serious consequences. Emphasize your commitment to safeguarding against any subtle or obvious acts of retaliation against the complainants. Make it clear that, as part of the follow-through to this meeting, complainants will be interviewed periodically to make sure that the disruptive behavior stops. At the end of the meeting, summarize key points and specify a plan for follow-up.

Follow Up

Remember the power of the written word. Write a summary letter of the meeting to the physician, and ask the physician to acknowledge that the summary is accurate.

Follow up and monitor progress as regular monitoring improves the chances for maintaining positive change. Tailor the follow-up plan to the nature and severity of the problems. Generally, follow-up meetings can be brief, but they should be held regularly. If you err here, do so by meeting more frequently than less frequently. We recommend that you meet at least once per month during the first 4 months postintervention. Then, if all is going well, meet once every 6 to 8 weeks for the remainder of the year. Do the following during these meetings:

- If problems persist, balance positive and negative feedback. Be specific regarding any criticisms or areas of needed improvement.
- Tell the physician when things are getting better. Remember that positive feedback is more powerful than negative feedback in influencing behavior.
- Summarize and agree on the immediate next steps.
- Confirm the next meeting date and place.
- Always encourage the physician.

DEALING WITH CRITICISM

It is difficult to be the target of another person's criticism. Whether you are the person orchestrating an intervention with a disruptive physician or the target of the intervention itself, the following general guidelines for dealing with criticism can be helpful:[21]

- See criticism as valuable information about how to do better, not as a personal attack.
- Don't react with defensiveness.
- If needed, ask to resume the meeting later, after you've had a cool-down period.
- See criticism as an opportunity to work together with the criticizer to solve a problem, not as an adversarial situation.

Additional guidelines for responding to criticism are outlined in Chapter 13.

Also of importance is the ability to respond appropriately when someone is upset. Following are some specific guidelines:[22]

- Remain silent and let them express their concerns.
- Thank the person and explain why you are glad they gave you this feedback.
- After listening, the first statement you make should specify your intent. Otherwise you risk losing your persuasive power. (Eg, "It is not my intent to upset you. It is my intent to _____ (fill in the blank.")
- Apologize for the problem. (Eg, "I am sorry that this problem has occurred.").
- Ask "What would you like me to do to fix this problem?"
- Say what you can do and what you cannot do.

- Promise to deal with the problem right away.
- Collect all the information you need.
- Correct the mistake as quickly as possible.
- Follow up to make sure that the other person is satisfied with your actions.

FINAL WORDS: IS YOUR JOB WORTH KEEPING?

If you are a disgruntled physician, it might be worth exploring the meanings of your discontent. On a superficial level, you probably feel that your distress is due to the incompetence of others—colleagues, nurses, or hospital administrators who simply do not hold up their end of the "bargains" that shape the quality of your professional life.

But it may also be the case that your distress signals deeper levels of ambivalence about your career that you need to honestly assess. Ask yourself:[23]

- Am I practicing the sort of medicine I love?
- Am I and my colleagues reasonably compatible?
- Does my practice suit my personality in terms of needs for affiliation/isolation, independence/collaboration?
- Do I live in the geographic area of the country that suits my needs?
- Can I imagine a practice or career circumstance that would soothe what ails me?
- What information do I need in order to discover if, indeed, the "grass is greener" in another professional milieu?

CONCLUSIONS

On an individual level, disruptive workplace behavior is symptomatic of distress and of the need for help. Disruptive behavior also signals an immediate need for a cohesive organizational response. Dealing with this problem can prove to be one of the most important and powerful formative events in the unfolding history of your career and of your organization.

REFERENCES–CHAPTER 9

1. Donaldson LJ. Doctors with problems in an NHS workforce. *BMJ.* 1994;308:1277–1282.

2. Springer E, Casale H. Hospitals and the disruptive health care practitioner—Is the inability to work with others enough to warrant exclusion? *Duquesne Law Review.* 1985;24:377.

3. Ryan KD, Oestreich DK. *Driving Fear Out of the Workplace,* 2nd ed. San Francisco, Calif: Jossey-Bass; 1998.

4. Gendel MH. Disruptive behaviors, personality problems, and boundary violations. In: Goldman L, Myers M, Dickstein L, eds. *The Handbook of Physician Health.* Chicago, Ill: American Medical Association; 2000:138–160.

5. Horty J. The disruptive physician. *Conn Med.* 1985;49:805–819.

6. Horty J, Barker M. Provisional conduct. In: *Medical Staff Leader Handbook.* Pittsburgh, Pa: Action Kit Publications; 1999:1–38.

7. Neff KE, Samoulis S, Widra L. Managing disruptive behavior in the hospital. Presented to: VHA Leadership Conference; April 16–19, 2000; Dallas, Texas.

8. VanKomen GJ. Troubled or troubling physicians: Administrative responses. In: Goldman L, Myers M, Dickstein L, eds. *The Handbook of Physician Health.* Chicago, Ill: American Medical Association; 2000:205–227.

9. Spector PE. Individual differences in the job stress process of health care professionals In: Firth-Cozens J, Payne R, eds. *Stress in Health Professionals: Psychological and Organisational Causes and Interventions.* New York, NY: John Wiley & Sons; 1999:33–42.

10. Brown RC. What sparks threats on the job? Forsyth Medicine/Business Coalition Meeting; September 10, 1999; Winston-Salem, NC.

11. Marcus IM. Harmony vs. discord in marriage: A view of physicians' marriages. *J of the Louisiana State Medical Society.* 1980;132:173–178.

12. Slaby R, Guerra N. Cognitive mediators of aggression in adolescent offenders. *Dev Psychol.* 1988;24:277–289.

13. Sotile WM, Sotile MO. Conflict management: Part 1. How to shape positive relationships in medical practices and hospitals. *The Physician Executive.* 1999;25:57–61.

14. Sotile WM, Sotile MO. Conflict management: Part 2. How to shape positive relationships in medical practices and hospitals. *The Physician Executive.* 1999;25:51–55.

15. Lowes R. Taming the disruptive doctor. *Med Econ.* 1998;5:67–68, 73–74,77–78, 80.

16. Pfifferling J-H. Managing the unmanageable: The disruptive physician. *Family Practice Management.* 1997;Nov/Dec:77–78, 83, 87–88, 90, 92.

17. Moore HL, Cangelosi JD, Gatlin-Watts RW. Seven spoonfuls of preventive medicine for sexual harassment in health care. *Health Care Supervisor.* 1998;17:1–9.

18. Baron R. Countering the effects of destructive criticism: The relative efficacy of four interventions. *J Appl Psychol.* 1990:75:3.

19. Sotile WM, Sotile MO. The angry physician: The temper-tantruming physician. *The Physician Executive.* 1996;22:30–34.

20. Sotile WM, Sotile MO. The angry physician: II. Managing yourself while managing others. *The Physician Executive.* 1996; 22:39–42.

21. Levinson H. Feedback to subordinates. I Addendum to the Levinson Letter. Waltham, Mass: Levinson Institute; 1992.

22. Barnard S. *Building Your Practice Through Effective Communication. Career Pathways in Urology.* American Urological Association: Atlanta, Ga; May 2000.

23. Cejka S. The best job may be the one you already have. *Med Econ.* 1998;5:31–32.

chapter 10

Listening and Communications Skills

"The three most important words for a successful relationship are communication, communication, and communication."

Anonymous

Communication is the link between your intentions and the outcomes of your efforts and the quality of your relationships. Some propose that communication is the relationship itself, since without it, a relationship is not possible.[1] Consider the important role that communication plays in your dealings with patients, colleagues, and loved ones.

With patients. When patients feel understood, they are more compliant, express greater levels of satisfaction with their medical care, respond more positively to medical care, and are more eager to modify their health behaviors in positive ways.[2] Specifically, a survey of 1,500 patients and physicians, conducted by the Bayer Institute for Health Care Communication, reported that patients who rated communications with their physicians as excellent were 4 times more likely to believe they had received excellent health care than those who did not highly rate their communications with their physicians.[3]

In a second noteworthy study, DiMatteo and colleagues[4] used data from physicians and patients participating in the Medical Outcomes Study to assess the influence of physicians attributes and practice styles on patients adherence. In a 2-year longitudinal study of 186 physicians and their patients, these researchers found that medication adherence was actually better among the patients of physicians who had busier practices (ie, those who saw more patients each week). But these busy physicians did other things that promoted the adherence: They made definite follow-up appointments with their patients, they were willing to answer all of the patients questions regarding the topic of care (eg, exercise), and they were willing to clarify the patients' questions. In other words, it was not time spent, *but the way the physicians managed their relationships with the patients,* that made the difference. The key was good communication.

In medical practice, absence of good communication fosters negative emotional outcomes. Research has shown that the poorer the patient–physician communication, the less satisfied the patient. And the more dissatisfied the patient is, the more likely it will be that he or she will be litigious. The Society for the Advancement of Education reported in 1997 that the primary reason patients with bad outcomes sued for malpractice was not the quality of care or medical negligence, it was how physicians talked to them.[5] In an article appearing in the June 27, 1994, issue of the *Archives of Internal Medicine,* Howard Beckman, MD, and colleagues reported that tensions in patient–physician relationships prompted 71% of malpractice lawsuit depositions.[6] Common themes reported by litigants included perceived physician unavailability, poor delivery of information, and physicians repeated failure to understand patients' concerns or those of their families.

Of course, communication is a two-way street, and it could be argued that patients need to be clearer in expressing their concerns. Stewart[7] indicated that 54% of patient problems and 45% of their concerns are missed in the interaction because physicians do not elicit them and patients do not offer appropriate information.

With colleagues. Throughout this book, we have established the fact that for all health care providers, effective workplace teamwork is a key to stress resilience and collegiality. We reiterate our observation that many physicians add significant complexity to their already stressful lives by failing to take responsibility for how they communicate with colleagues, nurses, and administrators. In a study of 882 physicians in the United Kingdom, burnout was more prevalent among those who felt insufficiently trained in communication and management skills.[8]

With loved ones. "He never listens to me!" "What does she want? All I do is work and worry, and now I have to hear her complaining that I don't care enough to listen. What a joke! I listen! What do I have to do to make her feel heard?"

In one form or another, this represents the most typical conversation heard in our counseling offices. And it's not always the man who is accused of not listening. These days, we almost as frequently encounter couples where it's the husband complaining that his overworked, driven wife falls short when it comes to their communication.

It has been proposed that, unfortunately, medical training teaches clinicians to value cultivating objective data more than cultivating relationships.[9] Excellent guidelines for patient–physician communication are offered in two books published by the American Medical Association, *Communicating with Your Patients: Skills for Building Rapport*[2] and *Physician-Patient Relations: A Guide to Improving Satisfaction.*[3] In this chapter, we draw material from these and other resources[10] to offer a set of communication guidelines that can improve relationships of all sorts. We intend for this chapter to be a primer on effective communication. As you review this material, you will likely be reminded of many points you already know but perhaps forget to practice. We hope that a careful reading will teach you a few new strategies that will make you a better, more effective communicator. The effective use of communication skills is a key to collaboration, collegiality, quality of patient care, and satisfying personal relationships.

CHARACTERISTICS OF GOOD COMMUNICATORS

When it comes to your communication style and effectiveness, how would you guess other people describe you? If you are truly a good communicator, people who know you would probably use phrases like:[3,11]

"He's always open to other people's ideas."

"I always know where she's coming from. I might not agree with her, but I do understand her point of view. She's very clear."

"She really seems interested in what you have to say."

"Even in a room full of people, when you talk with him he listens only to *you*."

"He's a really warm person."

"She seemed to be impacted by what I said, like she was *involved* in my concerns."

"You always feel on equal footing when you talk with him. He treats you with respect."

"She not only listens, she adds stuff to the conversation."

"I like the fact that he always answers the questions that I pose, or at least acknowledges them, even if he doesn't know the answer."

What, specifically, do good communicators do to earn such compliments? In the pages to follow, we discuss the skills shared by great communicators.

Be Assertive Rather than Passive or Aggressive

It is elucidating to think of communication coming in three possible "flavors:" passive, aggressive, and assertive. Olson and Olson[12] differentiated these communication styles in this way. Passive communication is characterized by an unwillingness to honestly share thoughts, feelings, or desires. This form of passivity is a barrier to collaboration or intimacy. Aggressive communication is characterized by blaming and accusatory actions. Often, aggression is signaled by language like "You always" or "You never," and it focuses on the negative characteristics of the person rather than the problem. Assertive communication involves asking clearly and directly for what one wants and being positive and respectful in one's communication.

In any two-person relationship, these three communication styles interact to create the various relationship outcomes outlined in Table 10-1.

Assertiveness is the ability to confidently and comfortably express your thoughts and feelings while still respecting the legitimate rights of others. Assertion is not continual confrontation but making a conscious choice about what to say, when to say it, how to say it, and to whom. Aggressiveness, on the other hand, is "that loud, forceful, often confrontational, way of trying to get what we want, even at the expense of others."[10 (p.9)]

The transactional differences between assertion and aggression can be quite subtle. For example, using the word *and* instead of *but* when offering criticism or differing opinion can make a tremendous difference. The word *but* tends to put the other person

TABLE   10-1

Communication Patterns and Their Effects

Communication Person A	Person B	Relationship Effect	Who wins?	Level of Intimacy or Collaboration
Passive	Passive	Devitalized	Both lose	Low
Passive	Aggressive	Dominating	I win, You lose	Low
Aggressive	Aggressive	Conflicted	Both lose	Low
Assertive	Passive	Frustrated	Both lose	Low
Assertive	Aggressive	Confrontational	Both lose	Low
Assertive	Assertive	Vital/Growing	Both win	High

Source: Olson DH, Olson AK. *Empowering Couples: Building on Your Strengths.* Minneapolis, Minn: Life Innovations, Inc.; 2000. Web site Life Innovations, Inc: www.lifeinnovations.com. Used with permission.

on the defensive because it tends to diminish the importance of what precedes it. Consider the following examples:

Aggressive: "I appreciate what you are saying, *but* if you'll hear me out, we will find a way to resolve this."

Assertive: "I appreciate what you are saying, *and* I think that if you'll hear me out, we will find a way to resolve this."

Aggressive: "Sure, your ideas make sense, *but* you need to hear my ideas."

Assertive: "Your ideas make sense to me, *and* I hope that my idea will make sense to you."

Show Warmth

Good communicators show positive regard for others. They freely and frequently hand out compliments like the following:[13]

"It took a lot of courage for you to. . ."
"You're always willing to help."
"You're always open to new ideas."
"I see improvement in. . ."
"We've worked hard on this."
"We came up with some good ideas."

Warmth is one of the most difficult interpersonal communication behaviors to learn. Warmth is displayed primarily in a nonverbal manner, through subtle facial and body signs, as well as gestures (small movements of the hand, brow, or eye). In our experience, the warmth that physicians may feel toward others often goes unexpressed or unnoticed, perhaps due to a lifetime of training that taught the benefits of remaining calm and keeping a "therapeutic distance" when dealing with emotional situations. Unfortunately, doing so puts physicians at risk of being perceived as cold, aloof, or intimidating. Use the following guidelines to ensure that you convey warmth:

- Relax the muscles of your face, forehead, and brow. Try not to frown or furrow your brow. Smile in a friendly manner
- Maintain comfortable eye contact. Providing eye contact juxtaposed with brief periods of looking away is best.
- Nod your head or show facial expressions that indicate you are listening.
- Position yourself to be eye level with the other person. Lean toward the other person slightly and give them your full attention.
- Maintain an open, receptive posture. Face the other person; do not cross your arms or otherwise indicated closedness to the other person.
- Gesture comfortably but do not point your finger or fidget as you listen or make your points.
- Use tones of voice and words that convey interest and compassion

If you want to improve the warmth factor in your communications, start by observing the communication style of someone whom you find to be warm. How do they act? What is their verbal tone? What is their body posture? What are their facial expressions?

Show Empathy

In his book, *Breaking Bad News: A Guide for Health Care Professionals*, oncologist and associate professor of medicine at the University of Toronto, Robert Buckman, MD,[15] reminds us that empathy is not a matter of what you *feel*. It's a matter of how you *behave*.

T A B L E 10-2

Keys to Respectful Communication With Patients

Do	Don't
Apologize if you kept the patient waiting	Act as though your time is more valuable than the patient's time
Acknowledge the patient prior to the exam	Simply start the examination
Use the patient's name	Refer to the patient as the "broken leg in Room 2"
If possible, demonstrate a knowledge of the patient's personal and family history	Act as though you have no history with the patient or his/her family
Tell the patient what you are going to do during the examination before doing it	Conduct the examination in silence
Sit, if possible	Stand over patient
Touch the patient's arm or shoulder while examining	Touch the patient only through tools like the stethoscope or tongue blade
Ask some open-ended questions	Use only "yes-or-no," or closed, questions
Listen intently to what the patient says	Tune out the patient while formulating your response to one of the patient's comments
Make appropriate eye contact	Chart while talking
Inquire about a range of patient concerns	Ignore the patient's feelings/fears
Apologize for and explain any interruption	Ignore the patient while attending to an interruption
Involve the patient in treatment options	Order the patient to do something

Sources: Summary of information from: Moise H. Physician-Patient Relations: *A Guide to Improving Satisfaction.* Chicago: American Medical Association, 1999; and O'Mara K. Communication and conflict resolution in emergency medicine. *Emergency Medicine Clinics of North America.* 1999 (May);17(2):451-459.

The key skill in conveying empathy is active listening that rests on tuning into the other's experience. This requires enough calm and receptivity that the subtle signs of feeling from another person can be received—the 90% or more of the emotional message that comes from nonverbal channels like tone of voice, gestures, facial expression, and the like.[16] See table 10-2 for some keys to respectful communication with patients.

But active listening does not mean repeating verbatim what others have told you. Quite the contrary: Parroting only irritates speakers, implying that you have not really processed what they have said or understood them. It is far better to choose your own words and respond in your own style.

Following are nine steps for communicating more empathically:[10 (pp. 126–127); 17]

1. Clear your head of distracting agendas. Focus on the person you are with.
2. Remind yourself to focus on your speaker. Tune into the speaker. Don't interrupt.
3. Attend to the other person's verbal and nonverbal messages. Tune in not only to the speaker's words but also look for what the speaker is saying nonverbally.
4. Ask yourself, "What does this person want me to hear?" The predominant theme of the speaker's message is the embryo for your empathic response.
5. Convey an empathic response. Summarize in your own words what you think the person is saying. Verbally reflect the speaker's feelings and the reason for them. Do not make any judgmental statement about what the speaker said.
6. Check to see if your empathic response was effective. Notice the speaker's response. Remember that "the purpose of being empathic is to make others feel relieved (that we understand them) and cared for (by our genuine interest in their situation)."[10 (p. 127)]
7. If the other person feels that you do not understand, explain that you want to and ask what points or feelings you seem to be missing.
8. If the other person says you do understand, ask what can be done to resolve the situation.
9. Even if you disagree with the speaker, it still is important to remember to validate his/her feelings.

In *The Patient's Story*, Smith and Engel use the mnemonic NURS to summarize key points to remember in order to increase your empathic impact:

- *Name the emotion.* This shows that you recognize what is being said. Example: "You sound worried about this."
- *Show that you Understand the patient's reaction:* "These are understandable concerns; I can see why you would be worried."

- *Show Respect for your patient and what he or she has been through:* "You've been through so much. I really admire how you and your family have coped."
- *Support the person and show that your relationship is a partnership:* "I want to help in any way I can. I believe that we can work together to solve this."

Listen

Few interpersonal skills are as powerful as listening. Listening involves the eyes, ears, and the heart. It is the key to establishing rapport and trust, to conveying compassion, and to influencing others.

Unfortunately, the busier or more rushed or stressed we get, the more we tend to suspend our use of effective listening skills. Listening is also the first skill to be abandoned when people become embroiled in conflict. Put simply: Stress and conflict have a way of clogging our ears. We focus on eliminating the source of our stress, especially if the stressor is another person, and ignore the many ways that our own behaviors may be perpetuating the situation or interchange that is stressing us in the first place.

Communication experts generally agree that any combination of the following factors predispose us to failed listening: if you have not been trained in effective listening skills; if you fail to concentrate on the other's point of view; and if your ego gets in the way—you focus exclusively on your own experience, ideas, jokes, goals, or so forth.

If you are to be an exceptional communicator, you have to develop the habit of spending as much time listening as you do talking or thinking about what you are planning to say. Remember the six guidelines for better listening summarized by the L-A-D-D-E-R mnemonic:[19]

1. *Look at the other person.* People don't trust someone who doesn't look at them. Attend to both the speaker's intent and content.
2. *Ask questions.* Asking appropriate question is an effective way to establish rapport with others. Avoid the tendency to launch into a "sales pitch" or a bout of dictating to another what he or she "should" think or do.[20] Remember: People support ideas that they agree with and help to shape,

especially if the idea relates to something they will derive benefit from.

It is most effective to use a combination of different types of questions. For example, closed-ended questions are good for discovering facts. (Examples: "Is this lab report up-to-date?" "Are you on call this weekend?").

Open-ended questions, on the other hand, encourage others to speak about themselves or their experiences. (Examples: "How's it going for you since you joined the practice?" "How is your family doing since the school year started?")

A simple way to remember the difference between open-ended and closed-ended questions follows: Who, where, and when begin closed-ended questions. What, why, and how begin open-ended questions.

3. *Don't interrupt.* Let others finish sentences and ideas. The quickest way to assure that another person will be defensive about what you have to say is to interrupt them when it's their turn to speak.

As simple as it may seem, a key to effective communication is paying the speaker the courtesy of letting him or her finish what they are saying without interruption. This is a difficult one for many physicians, perhaps due to habits borne of patient–physician interactions in which physicians maintain control of the conversation for the sake of getting important information covered in the typically brief time allotted for the consultation. You may believe that in this age of heightened awareness, physicians are better than they used to be at this. In fact, studies of physician–patient interaction indicate that the number of seconds physicians allow patients to speak before they interrupted the conversations expanded from 18 seconds in 1984, to only 23 seconds in 1999.[21,22] In only 2% of these conversations did the physicians return to address their patients' original agendas.

4. *Don't change the subject.* Interrupting another is bad enough. But abruptly changing the subject can be downright discourteous, and it can slaughter rapport with the speaker. This is a mistake to be avoided in any relationship.

In her book, *Claiming Power in Doctor-Patient Talk,* author Nancy Ainsworth-Vaughn[23] reported on the different communication styles shown by male and female physicians during patient interactions. One finding was that male physicians moved to a new topic without getting the patient's verbal agreement almost as often as they got patients' agreement. (They got permission to switch topics only 1.4 times for every 1 time they switched topics without getting permission.) Female physicians, on the other hand, sought patient agreement to switch topics 5 times for every 1 time they abruptly switched topics without the patient's consent (ratio of 5:1). Examples of both styles of communicating follow.

Example of abruptly changing the topic with seeming insensitivity to the patient:

Patient: "I'm worried about taking this medicine long-term."

Physician: "Okay. Don't forget what I told you about exercising. Ms Johnson will get you scheduled for a follow-up."

Example of getting the patient's agreement before changing topics:

Patient: "I'm worried about taking this medicine long-term."

Physician: "What are your concerns?" (Listens attentively.) "I can appreciate your concerns. I, too, hope that you will eventually be able to lessen or stop this medicine. There are some things that might increase the odds that you will be able to discontinue the medicine sooner. Would you like to learn what those are?"

(Patient nods her head, indicating that she is open to switching topics.)

Physician: "Great. Let's start by discussing how exercising regularly might help you."

We fully realize that in today's environment, even physicians who are great communicators and compassionate individuals face the demand to function efficiently. You must assess the patient's problems, deliver your interventions, and move on to the next patient.

But remember that common courtesies of the sort that build positive communication do not have to take inordinate amounts of time. Be careful to curb any tendency to act authoritarian when communicating with peers or other equals. Remember that "Expressing opinions is not telling others what to do, but giving them the benefit of your point of view."[10 (p. 171)]

To express opinions without alienating the other person, get the consent of the other before expressing your opinions. Avoid generating feelings of hostility or resistance by asking if they are interested in hearing your viewpoint. Make allowances for the uniqueness of others, and avoid being dogmatic when expressing your opinions. Show consideration for others by avoiding strong phrases like "It should be clear to you that this is the thing to do." Rather, when offering your opinions, include one of the following phrases, which convey respect of the other's right to accept or reject your ideas: "Do you think this suggestion might help in your situation?" "What do you think?" "How does this sound to you?" "Can you see adapting any of these ideas to your situation?" Include the rationale for your viewpoint. Offer the reasons you are using to defend your position.

5. *Curb your Emotions.* Hinz[2] reported that Barry Enger, MD, medical director of the Northwest Center for Physician–Patient Communication, suggests five emotion-handling skills for dealing with upset people:

- *Reflect:* Name the emotion the other person is showing so they see that you are paying attention: "You seem to be really bothered by this."
- *Validate:* Explain that you understand why the other is upset and show that you are concerned: "I can understand your being angry about my being late." Or, you might choose to say something like this: "I can understand that anyone who feels they've been double-crossed would be upset."
- *Support:* Offer both verbal and nonverbal responses that ease the immediate stress. "I'd like to help" (accompanied by placing your hand on the other's shoulder).
- *Partnership:* Offer the request to move forward. "I wonder what we could do to get beyond this. What would help?"
- *Respect:* Honor the other person and respect his or her autonomy. "I want you to know that despite this difficulty, I hold you in high regard."

When communicating about emotional issues—particularly if the other person is upset—it is a good guideline to stick with "I" statements: those that describe your feelings or intentions in reacting to the other person. Avoid any destructive labeling statement and try to focus on how you might work together to improve or rectify this situation. Ignore threats and never state or imply any yourself. Try to keep the conversation focused on the point at hand, which is to resolve this difficult situation or, at minimum, to soothe the other person's ruffled feathers. Acknowledge the other person's argument, whether or not it seems valid to you, and reiterate your own point.[17]

The major faults of the worst listeners span two ends of a reactive continuum: They either overreact or underreact to what the speaker says.

Curb your emotional reactions to what the speaker says. Don't interrupt, jump to conclusions, or show nonverbal indicators of impatience, boredom, or distress in responding to what you hear.

6. *Respond.* Show some reaction other than impersonal note taking. Remember: Your job is to listen and reflect interest and understanding of the speaker. When it's your turn to talk, you are more likely to have an attentive listener if you manage to listen without alienating the other by reacting negatively to certain of his words or phrases. Be aware of your tone of voice[20]—watch for a rise in your voice when you become annoyed, speak to others as a peer rather than a parent, and avoid threats and scare tactics.

Be Specific

Two factors that help foster good communication require particular self-awareness: (1) You must specify what you think, feel, need, or want and (2) you must do so in a manner that is congruent. Make sure that your body language, tone of voice, facial expression, and word choices align to congruently convey your message. Also, speak in specific, concrete terms.[20] Following are a few examples.

Congruent and Specific: "I'd really appreciate it if we could agree to meet again next week—any evening other than Wednesday—rather than waiting until our next scheduled meeting time, which is more than a month away."

Vague: "Well, a month is a long way off. We still have lots to resolve."

Congruent and Specific: "I'll finish rounds between 6:30 and 7:15, so I'd like for us to agree to meet at the restaurant at 8:00."

Vague: "I'll get there as soon as I can."

Self-Disclose with Discretion

Effective communicators balance soliciting information from others with giving information about themselves. Think about it. If you are like most people, the "great communicators" you know are people who at once show an interest in you and let you in on relevant information about themselves.

This does not mean that you have to tell every patient or colleague the intimate details of your life. But offering appropriate information about yourself creates the opportunity to build a sense of common ground. Most of us share similar if not common experiences. We struggle with frustrations about work and concerns about loved ones. We have opinions of world events or the latest ball game that has made the news, and so on. Often, we have had personal experiences relevant to the topic of conversation. If shared appropriately, such information can greatly enhance rapport. The following examples show how appropriate self-disclosure might be worked into conversations:

- *In patient care:* "I know that the news of a diagnosis is upsetting, Mr Jones. I've been there myself. I want you to know that I will try my best to help you with this."
- *When dealing with a colleague:* "Sure, we can end this meeting a little early. Glad to hear that you'll be able to make it to your daughter's ball game. How long has she played? (Listen attentively.) That's great. I've got great memories myself—and a few regrets—about my own family life when my kids were that age."
- *With a loved one:* "Joan, you know that I love you. I'm sorry that what I did upset you. It's just that I've been so stressed lately. I'm really worried about what's happening at the hospital. I know I seem angry about it, but I'm also scared. I don't know where this is going."

Use Humor Appropriately

Great communicators do more than listen and speak; they attend to others in a manner that creates a comfortable interchange. Appropriate use of humor can be a great help here. The emphasis is on "appropriate." Be aware that wit and dry humor are often interpreted as sarcasm. Be sensitive to others' feelings about being teased or embarrassed. Safest of all is to use self-depreciating humor. Pointing out your own foibles is a great way to show others that you are approachable.

Select Positive Words

Another strategy for setting a positive tone used by great communicators is to use positive words to convey points. Communications expert Stephanie Barnard makes several specific recommendations in this regard:[20]

- Avoid using negative words such as "don't", "won't," "didn't," or "can't."
- Replace "You better" with "I suggest."
- Speak carefully when delegating.
  Poor: "You try to handle this, but let me check it before it goes out."
  Better choice: "I know that you can handle this. Let me know if I can help."

Match the Pace of the Person to Whom You Are Speaking

As we mentioned in our discussion of disruptive colleagues, it is important to adjust your communication to match the mood and style of your partner. Especially when dealing with others who are upset, it is important to pace your tone, body movements, and emotional expression. Your facial mimicry, vocal synchrony (volume, speech rhythm, tone), and movement coordination when conversing with another person will either increase their emotional state, reduce it, or convert it to a different emotional frame.[17] Start by matching the other's state, then gradually begin modeling a more adaptive response set.

Examples:

> *Poor:* "Whoa, John! Calm down. Things can't possibly be that bad. Come on. . . let's just mellow out and discuss this rationally."

> *Better:* "I hear you, John. (Standing to match John's tense stance.) It makes absolute sense to me that you are really angry about this. (John nods and relaxes a bit.) Help me to better understand exactly what happened." (Listening with arms crossed to match John's similar stance.)

> (Eventually) "Listen (more calmly). Why don't we go sit in the conference room and discuss this in detail."

Check Your Hearing

At risk of preaching to the choir, indulge two laymen as we offer you this reminder: If you often find yourself the target of comments like "You never listen!" or "I told you that, didn't you listen?" consider this: It may be that you listen just fine but that you can't hear! Over 40 million Americans suffer from hearing impairments. It might be worth having your hearing checked before deciding that you are a poor communicator.

CONCLUSIONS

The rudimentary rules of good communication are, indeed, worth revisiting periodically. By practicing the essentials of clear communication, you can enhance your effectiveness in any realm.

We close with a checklist of questions and factors drawn from the works of the various communications experts cited in this chapter. Periodically reviewing this list can help to keep you aware of your communication style.

- What kind of climate do I create?
- How do I see myself as a communicator?
- Given my communication style, how must others experience me?
- Am I a willing listener?
- Do I draw out other's point of view?
- Do I concentrate on trying to understand the speaker rather than spend time preparing my next remark?

- Before agreeing or disagreeing, do I check to make sure I do understand what others mean?
- Do I try to summarize points of agreement or disagreement?
- Do I try to ask questions that result in more information than yes or no answers?
- Do I try to encourage others to participate in the discussion?
- Do I guard against assuming I know what others mean by asking questions to assure understanding?
- Do I "listen" for others' feelings as they are speaking?
- When another person's feelings are hurt, do I respond with caring?

I am willing to commit to mindfully practice the following two communication skills this week:

At home: 1._____

2._____

At work: 1._____

2._____

REFERENCES—CHAPTER 10

1. Stuart GW, Sundeen SJ. *Principles and Practice of Psychiatric Nursing,* 5th ed. St Louis, Mo: Mosby; 1995.
2. Hinz CA. *Communicating with Your Patients: Skills for Building Rapport.* Chicago, Ill: American Medical Association; 2000.
3. Moise H. *Physician-Patient Relations: A Guide to Improving Satisfaction.* Chicago, Ill: American Medical Association; 1999.
4. DiMatteo MR, Sherbourne CD, Hays RD, Ordway L, Dravitz RL, McGlynn EA, Kaplan S, Rogers WH. Physicians' characteristics influence patients' adherence to medical treatment: Results from the Medical Outcomes Study. *Health Psychol.* 1993;12:93–102.
5. Society for the Advancement of Education. Communication skills cut malpractice risk. *USA Today.* October 1997.
6. Beckman H, Markakis K, Suchman A, Frankel R. The doctor-patient relationship and malpractice: Lessons from plaintiff depositions. *Arch Intern Med.* 1994a;154:1365–1369.
7. Stewart M. Effective physician-patient communication and health outcomes: A review. *Can Med Assoc J.* 1995;152:1423–1432.
8. Ramirez AJ, Graham J, Richards MA, Cull A, Gregory WM. Mental health of hospital consultants: The effects of stress and satisfaction at work. *Lancet.* 1996;347:724–728.
9. Suchman A, Markakis K, Beckman H, Frankel R. A model of empathic communication in the medical interview. *JAMA.* 1997; 277:678–682.
10. Balzer-Riley JW. *Communication in Nursing,* 3rd ed. St. Louis, Mo: Mosby; 1996.
11. Burgoon JK, Pfau M, Parrott R, Birk T, Coker R, Burgoon M. Relational communication, satisfaction, compliance-gaining strategies, and compliance in communication between physicians and patients. *Commun Monogr.* 1987;54(2):307–324.
12. Olson DH, Olson AK. *Empowering Couples: Building on Your Strengths.* Minneapolis, Minn: Life Innovations, Inc; 2000.
13. Berent IM, Evans RL. *The Right Words: The 350 Best Things to Say to Get Along with People.* New York, NY: Warner; 1992.
14. O'Mara K. Communication and conflict resolution in emergency medicine. *Emerg Med Clin North Am.* 1999;17:451–459.

15. Buckman R. *How to Break Bad News: A Guide for Health Care Professionals.* Baltimore, Md: Johns Hopkins University Press; 1992.

16. Goleman D. *Emotional Intelligence.* New York, NY: Bantam Books; 1995.

17. Weisinger H. *Anger at Work.* New York, NY: William Morrow and Co; 1995.

18. Smith RC, Engel G. *The Patient's Story.* Boston, Mass: Little, Brown & Company; 1996.

19. Nightengale E. *Listening* [audiotape series]. Niles, Ill: Nightengale-Conant Corp; 1995.

20. Beckman H, Markakis K, Suchman A, Frankel R. Getting the most from a 20-minute visit. *Am J Gastroenterol.* 1994b;89:662–664.

21. Barnard S. Building your practice through effective communication. Workshop presented to: Career Pathways in Urology, American Urological Association Annual Meeting; May, 2000; Atlanta, Ga.

22. Marvel M, Epstein R, Flowers K, Beckman H. Soliciting the patients' agenda: Have we improved? *JAMA.* 1999;281:283–287.

23. Ainsworth-Vaughn N. *Claiming Power in Doctor-Patient Talk (Oxford Studies in Sociolinguistics).* Oxford: Oxford University Press; 1998.

11

Coping With Change

"Whether things will be better if they are different I do not know,
but that they will have to be different if they are to become better,
that I do know."

George Christoph Lichtenberg
18th century writer[1]

One quality of resilient people is flexibility. They respond to
change with a combination of open-mindedness and self-
appraisal. Their honest self-assessment leads to action as they
concentrate their attention on the opportunities that come with
unexpected, unwanted changes. They pause and ask, "Now that
this has happened, what do I need to do next to assure continued
success?" They choose the future over the past and work to make
their new normal as good as it can be, without wasting energy on
guilt, blame, or criticism.[2] That's a lot easier said than done.

In truth, of course, not everyone manages to glide through
changes. Whether dealing with professional or personal change,
we sometimes react with a combination of dread, terror, anger, or
passive–aggressive resistance. Often, a roller coaster of poorly
managed reactions adds unnecessary complexity to the already
formidable task of coping with change.

This chapter will shed light on a number of strategies used by
those resilient types who manage change well. We focus on concepts and skills that can be helpful in coping with any type of
change, including family challenges, work transitions, or personal
lifestyle modifications.

BE REALISTIC: ANY CHANGE IS STRESSFUL

Many of the resilient physicians we know suffer from the strain of
a surprising, hidden stressor: The cumulative effects of the multi-
tude of wanted, *positive* changes that fill their lives. In addition to

acclimating to their demanding work-life balancing act, these exceptional people also tend to fervently pursue their dreams. They build vacation homes; open businesses outside of medicine; take on new, stimulating projects; and generally satisfy their penchant for high levels of stimulation. In so doing, they dodge the "hunkering-down" stress trap we talked about previously. But they make the mistake of underestimating the wear-and-tear effect that constant change can beget.

It's a simple truth: *Any* change is stressful. Both wanted and unwanted change requires that you adjust; therefore, both cause stress.

On the broadest level, change is stressful because it requires that we delve into as-yet uncharted territory. If the new territory comes about due to a positive change (like starting your practice, adding to your family, or retiring on schedule), feelings of joyful anticipation are likely to coat your stress responses. But make no mistake about it, the process of "finding your way" around this new territory does, indeed, elevate your baseline levels of stress. For this reason, choosing to control your lifestyle so that, where possible, you sequence change is advisable. More about this later.

It goes without saying that unwanted change is stressful. At such times, we tend to focus on questions that reflect our fears:[3] What does this change mean to me or to us? How will this impact our lives? What will now be expected of me? Will any positive come from this change?

The anxieties that underlie such questioning can lead to attempted solutions that simply complicate how you cope with change. Stress-hardy copers avoid these mistakes:

- Digging in and resisting the change
- Striking out at whomever or whatever is demanding or symbolizing the change
- Reluctantly accepting that change is necessary but dispassionately going about the adjustment process
- Giving up when faced with unexpected twists in the path of adjusting
- Soothing anxieties by focusing on illusions of control

This last mistake warrants elaboration.

Coping and Control

When do you feel best about yourself? When are you most at ease, self-confident, and relaxed? Most people answer such questions by describing relationships or situations in which they feel a sense of control. On the other hand, most people find that the hardest aspect of coping with change is dealing with any actual or perceived loss of control caused by the change. For this reason, gaining or maintaining a sense of control seems to be a key to managing the stress of change.

Maintaining a sense of control in the face of imposed changes is an especially difficult task for individuals who have an external locus of control. Locus of control[4] refers to beliefs about whether one is in control of the world or subject to control by the world. *Internals* believe they are largely in control of what happens to them. *Externals* believe they have little control over what happens and are fatalistic. When facing unwanted changes, externals are more stressed and more prone to depression than internals.[5] When faced with organizational constraints, role ambiguity, and role conflict at work, externals also report higher levels of distress, more job dissatisfaction, and greater work anxiety.[6,7]

The methods we use to try to soothe the anxiety that comes with unwanted changes often backfire. For example, you might choose to overfocus on some issue, task, or goal in the wake of the change. As we have explained, doing this allows us to *act as though* we are in control.

> "We believe that if we can just argue a single point loudly enough, or manage a single issue perfectly enough, or pursue a single goal relentlessly enough, then our anxiety about the larger changes we are facing will disappear."[8 (p. 116)]

If managed appropriately, this is not necessarily a bad coping strategy. The key is to chose your targets wisely. Focus on healthy choices, those that increase your sense of control or promote overall stress hardiness. For example, you might increase your sense of control by learning more about the new territory that comes with the change. Your child's adolescence, the administration of managed care contracts, or a new computer program might be examples here. Another strategy is using tried-and-true stress management behaviors like exercising or meditating, strategies that help you create a sense of control on any given day.

To be avoided are strategies like digging in your heels and arguing a minor point, simply for the sake of satisfying your need to control *something* during this uncontrollable time. Doing so will typically create more problems to deal with. For example, we once consulted with a medical group that was suffering from seriously diminished cash flow after having agreed to several deeply discounted managed care contracts. Morale in the group was quite low, and the managed care movement was the open target of the group's discontent. But the managed care contracts, *per se*, were not the true culprits causing this group's cash flow problems. The true culprit was several senior physicians who reacted negatively to this unwanted change. Sick and tired of "outside forces telling us how to practice medicine," several highly productive members of this group practice tacitly cooperated in a quiet, passive–aggressive rebellion that simply served to complicate their own plight. This "rebellion" came in the form of their refusal to expeditiously provide diagnoses of patients following routine office visits. On average, there was a 45-day delay between the point of contact with a patient and when the physician checked the diagnosis on the form that had to be submitted to the insurance company in order to get reimbursement for the office visit. When confronted with this fact, one of the group's senior partners admitted,

> "I'm so fed up with the paperwork these managed care companies require of us that I guess I no longer discriminate between which of their demands are reasonable and which are unreasonable. It literally takes only about 3 seconds to scan the sheet they provide and check the appropriate diagnosis. Refusing to do it is symbolic, and it feels sorta good—like fighting back. Of course, it also falls in the category of shooting ourselves in the foot."

ACCEPT THAT CHANGE IS INEVITABLE

We have noticed a common characteristic of individuals, couples, and medical organizations that struggle, rather than cope well: The people involved are surprised and dismayed when faced with repeated demands to change. It is as though they believe they should be allowed to "finally get it right"—the right balance, the right relationship dynamics, the right levels of professional productivity—then be left alone. Inevitably, of course, yet *another* unexpected demand upsets their world.

Whether you are facing another family problem, another developmental stage of life, another paradigm shift at work, or another health concern, learning to accept the inevitability of change and to frame change as an opportunity rather than a punishment is a key factor in avoiding the "double-crossed" syndrome outlined in Chapter 1. It helps to bear in mind that change comes in many flavors.

RECOGNIZE THE FLAVORS OF CHANGE

We have proposed that the stressors in medical training and medical family life fall into three broad categories[9] borrowed from the work of child psychologist David Elkind.[10] This taxonomy can also be used to highlight the various flavors of change we all encounter.

Anticipated But Unavoidable

Many of the changes that stress us are predictable, distressing, but predictable. A life in medicine comes with certain stressful guarantees:

- Medical school and residency will involve grueling work and study and the likelihood of having to relocate at some point in the course of your training.
- Family life will consist of an ever-evolving series of transitions driven by developmental changes in your relationships and for each of you individually.
- Exposure to the pain, suffering, and death of others will take its toll.
- Once training is completed, the new challenge will be to manage time pressures, financial pressures, and/or institutional pressures to produce more, and more, and more.
- Medical and communication technology developments will demand that you continue to update your skills and education, again, and again, and again.
- The ever-changing rules and regulations that interfere with physician autonomy will relentlessly continue.
- Life in medicine will require that you deal with ever-changing relationship dynamics (eg, in physician–physician, physician–patient, physician–administrator, physician–nurse, and physician–staff relationships).

- Periodic changes in the players who comprise your department, your practice, or your most valued work team are likely.

Even clearly anticipated changes like these are difficult to endure. But what gets toxic are the changes that fall into the next two categories.

Unanticipated and Unavoidable

Here, the surprises begin. Many of these stressors could actually be described as "I sort of anticipated this, but I had no idea coping with this would be so bad."

- The unprecedented academic challenges that come in the course of medical education.
- The backlog of debt that may greet you once medical training is completed.
- The role strains that may stretch the fiber of your marriage.
- The "physician bashing" that has become the rage of recent years.
- The ever-escalating costs of operating a medical practice.
- The often frustrating, sometimes violent attitudes of patients toward both the physician and his or her family.
- Repeated bouts of questioning and reappraisal of your work–family balance.
- Changes in stamina levels that come earlier in the aging process than you anticipated.
- The "surprise" that, rather than having one job, you are likely to end up combining several different areas of career involvement: clinician, consultant, teacher, medical politician, and businessperson.
- The stages of disillusionment with medicine and with your marriage.

Finally, come those changes caused by choices, not happenstance. These changes cause stress that medical families tend to hold each other accountable for, stress that may drain their collective energies.

Anticipated, Potentially Avoidable, But Not Avoided

These are the types of changes that may lead to disillusionment and self-questioning. We emphasize that the following list is *not intended* to describe physicians in general. Remember that these changes are avoidable. Indeed, most of the stress-hardy physicians we know work hard to avoid or correct these mistakes. Included here are such factors as:

- The string of life changes that may result from excessive ambitiousness.
- The burden of debt that may result from excessive materialism.
- The endless process of creating and re-creating one's professional life that may be fueled by competitiveness.
- Loss of one's ability to simply relax and enjoy life.
- Getting stuck in the attitude of needing to control others.
- Changing from a kind and caring person to one who is filled with hostility and cynicism.
- Losing one's ability to maintain a reasonable pace in daily living. Becoming someone who is stuck in the habit of constantly rushing, even when there is really no need to do so.

Continuous and Discontinuous Change

Consultant Ernie Lawson offered a simple but helpful way to think of change:[11]

"If you place a frog in a pot of cold water, then put the pot on a hot stove, the frog will happily swim around. It won't notice the subtle changes in the water's rising temperature until it is too late, and the heated water kills it.

If you place a frog into a pot of boiling water, however, the shock of the change will alarm the frog and it will jump out."

In the first instance, the increments in the change process are so small that they go unnoticed. This is called *continuous change*. This is the sort of change that gradually creeps into your life, one step at a time, and each step seems inconsequential in the moment. Herein may lie those subtle changes that erode morale, motivation, love, friendship, or one's physical health.

The second instance is an example of *discontinuous change.* Here, change is accompanied by the clear alarm that something big is happening. This type of change occurs when a loved one has an affair, a colleague attacks you in a fit of anger, or your perspective on life is abruptly altered by your own unwanted diagnosis. This is the sort of change that slaps us into paying attention and leads us to look back and notice subtle signs that the change was coming. We lament "If only I'd seen this coming earlier, I would have changed my course!"

In one way or another, resilient people make it a habit to regularly ask themselves, "If I suddenly face an unwanted change, what would I beg for a second chance to do more or less of?" Bob was a case in point.

Bob is a physician in our community who is revered by his colleagues, patients, and family. In response to our asking if he had a secret to his success, he told us this story:

"I can't say that I have a secret. But if you're asking whether I do something out of habit that helps me stay on track, the answer is yes. It's simply this: Every day, I take Hawthorne Road as I drive to work. When I pass the stop light at Knollwood and Hawthorne, I let it serve as a cue to me to play a 'What-If' game with myself. I ask, 'What if when I get to the office today, my two key people, Jane and Nancy, say to me 'We quit. We're going to work for someone else.' What would I beg them to give me a second chance to do more or less of, just to get them to stay?'

On my way home each evening when I pass that same intersection at Knollwood and Hawthorne, I go through a similar 'What-If' exercise, this time about my wife, Karen. I ask, 'What if when I get home Karen says to me, 'I don't love you anymore; I love someone else. What would I beg her to give me another chance to do more or less of, just to get her to stay?'

Thank goodness nothing dramatic has ever *really* happened in any of these relationships. But I can't help but believe that this little mental exercise might have nudged me to make small adjustments along the way that helped keep me on track. Those people—my office staff and my wife—they make my life possible. Those relationships have been worth working hard to preserve and protect."

OPERATIONALIZE YOUR WORRIES

If you are like most people, you start to worry when change hits. Some of us let worrying turn to obsessive rumination about worst-case scenarios that then fuel free-floating anxiety and distress.

Of course, it makes sense to do what you realistically can do to keep the worst-case scenario from materializing. But we often surprise participants in our change management seminars with this next piece of advice: When facing unwanted change, it is more fruitful to use your energy to focus in detail on exactly what is worrying you and then to develop an action plan that specifies how you will cope, if the worst happens. This recommendation flies in the face of the homespun advice to "try not to worry." Indeed, we find it helpful to take control of the worrying process that otherwise becomes an unwanted, obsessive endeavor.

Spending energy trying to ward off the worst-case scenario is sort of like asking yourself *not* to think about a white bear. The only way to accomplish this is to think about the bear and then try to cancel out the thought. Of course, in the process, you just thought about it.

Our worst-case scenarios typically have to do with things that are totally out of our control. By operationalizing the worry and developing an action plan for dealing with that scenario, you create a cognitive shift that may leave you feeling at least a modicum more in control.

Often, this syndrome can be broken if you ask yourself the following series of questions: Exactly what am I worrying about? What is the worst thing that can happen as result of this? What would I do then?

USE CHANGE AS AN OPPORTUNITY

Even a change of crisis proportions can be a healthy turning point for an individual, couple, family, or organization. The key is to let the change lead to healthy choices that align your behaviors and your values. Change is an opportunity to clarify your values and readjust your behaviors to live more in harmony with what you truly think, feel, need, or want.[12] Given the change you are facing, what is a goal that you can work toward? What are the stabilizing factors in your life?

DON'T ADD FUEL TO THE FIRE

"Now that this has happened, I'm tempted to just wipe the slate clean and start all over."

Whether dealing with the aftermath of a lost romance, a career setback, or other forms of unwanted change, it may be tempting to "throw in the towel" and start all over. The classic example is when someone reacts to the stress of a marital separation by introducing further unnecessary changes into his or her life.

"Wiping the slate clean and starting over can be an effective stress management strategy. However, first give yourself time to absorb the blow and the stress of the major change you are facing. Then, when the dust of your initial emotional reactions settles, look clearly at your options."[8 (p. 118)]

PRACTICE "CHANGE PROPHYLAXIS"

In *Beat Stress Together*, we called attention to the wisdom of exercising choice to control your lifestyle when choosing is possible.

"Don't jump at every opportunity that your Big Life presents. When possible, be selective and respectful of yourself and your loved ones in timing major changes. Pause before accepting an opportunity to change, even if the change is positive and exciting. Ask yourself whether the prices you will pay adjusting to the change are too high for you or for your loved ones. Be sure to ask loved ones how they feel about any change that you are considering."[8 (p. 117)]

We further advise that, if you do say no to an opportunity to change, frame the decision in a way that is self-affirming. Choose to view the decision as an indication of maturity, good judgment, wisdom, or commitment to maintaining a reasonably balanced lifestyle. And seek support for this decision from trusted friends and loved ones.

RESPECT EACH OTHER'S PACE

Change is stressful. But when the other people in your life resist joining in your style of reacting to change, the results can be infuriating. At a time when you most need supportive collaboration (a key to stress hardiness), you may find yourself at odds with those around you.

University of Rhode Island psychologist James Prochaska and his colleagues offered a way of understanding one's own and others' change processes.[13] Prochaska proposes that we tend to progress through predictable stages when changing any health behavior. In our own work, we have noted that both medical organizations and couples benefit from conceptualizing their change processes in these same terms.

In *precontemplation,* we have no intention of changing. We find ways to rationalize our continuing old ways, and we may be annoyed by others who either encourage us to change or who themselves embrace certain changes.

During *contemplation,* we begin to consider that we may need to change, but we are not yet ready to actually do anything different. We may decide to hear others out as they describe the pros and cons of changing, read articles or books regarding the topic in focus, and discuss the issues related to changing. But we are not yet ready to actually commit to making any specific change.

Preparation begins when we decide that we will take action in the next few months. Now we may begin experimenting with very small changes in the targeted area.

Action comes next. Here we begin to make definite changes in the area of concern. The first 6 months of actually changing tend to be quite awkward. Further input from others about *why* we should persist in our change efforts tends to be aggravating rather than helpful at this stage. Instead, what is needed is help to implement the change that you are committed to making.

According to Prochaska, after approximately 6 months of living with our changes, we enter *maintenance.* The work here is to prevent relapses into old ways and avoid overreacting to slips.

Bearing these stages of change in mind can help guide your own efforts to cope with change and also guide you as you try to help others do the same.

HOW TO HELP OTHERS COPE WITH CHANGE

Unmanaged or poorly managed change can wreak havoc in any organization or relationship. Whether a medical community, medical practice, or family, when a relationship system encounters disorganized change, predictable problems develop. Consultant Elizabeth Harper Neeld[3] pointed out that, at such times, teamwork, harmony, and productivity are threatened by a number of factors, including but not limited to the following:

- Unfocused behavior
- Confusion, lack of concentration, and impaired performance
- Anger, upset, and emotional outbursts
- Wasted energy exploring details of "what if" scenarios
- Lack of cooperation
- Whining and complaining
- Romanticizing the past
- In work settings: Rumors regarding negative consequences of the change becoming rampant
- In work settings: Increased absenteeism, tardiness, accidents
- In work settings: Decreased productivity
- Lack of cooperation

Reactions like these can splinter relationships at the very time when collaboration and caring connection are most needed. This quandary is worsened when, as is inevitably the case, different members of a relationship are at different stages in the change process outlined earlier. Amik and Ockene[14] outlined practical guidelines for soliciting and offering support through the various stages of change.[15]

1. Precontemplators
   - Ask for help in identifying ways that you might be defensive about making needed changes.
   - Tell supporters what would help you to change in the targeted area.
   - Ask for encouragement to cope in adaptive ways.

2. Contemplators
   - Ask for empathy and understanding about your issues relative to the targeted change.
   - Seek out and share information, awareness, observations, and personal experiences related to the targeted change.
   - Ask for help in noting messages and activities that increase awareness of the targeted change and its potential impact on you and/or your organization or relationships.

■ Ask for help in noting benefits of changing and information regarding how the targeted change might be implemented.

■ Ask for encouragement to change.

3. During Preparation

■ Announce a date or plan for making the targeted change.

■ Accept that changing is difficult.

■ Create a list of do's and don'ts that will help you to cope with the change.

4. During Action

■ Ask for and offer others support, encouragement, and, where possible, participation in the change.

■ Ask for and offer cooperation with whatever modifications in your lifestyle or working style might be required for positive coping with the change. For example, if you are taking action to improve your health, ask for cooperation from loved ones as you remove alcohol or tobacco products or unhealthy foods from your home. If you are undergoing a major change at work, ask for help from colleagues and loved ones in whatever areas might facilitate your ability to cope with the change.

■ Focus on positively reinforcing interactions. Solicit reminders of past successes in changing. Provide yourself with rewards for accomplishing incremental changes.

■ Avoid guilt induction.

■ Encourage and support expression of feelings regarding the change process.

■ Try to view the new behaviors that come with the change in a positive light.

■ Organize and/or participate in support groups or services related to the change. For example, you might seek out specialized training related to the skills needed to cope with the consequences of the change.

5. During Maintenance

■ Accept that your task now is to grow accustomed to the new life or work "territory" created by the change.

- Remember that everyone impacted by the change (including you!) will still need support.
- Organize support systems that will offer encouragement at times of floundering in the change-adjustment process.
- Help someone else cope with the change.
- Remember that no one changes with complete comfort and success. Normalize the fact that "slips" and lapses are part of the change process.
- Flag the first 2 months post-change as being the time that carries the highest risk of relapse into old behaviors.
- Be realistic about environmental, emotional, and interpersonal cues for problems in coping with the change.
- Block guilt-inducing ways of thinking or acting.

CONCLUSIONS

Coping with change is made easier if you are convinced that the pain of changing will be less than the pain of staying the same.[1] Taking control of your reactions to change always requires a commitment to EEM and accepting the fact that coping with change requires consistent and mindful effort. As the old saying goes, "If it was easy, everyone would do it."

Special coping challenges come when physicians react to the changing medical marketplace by merging practices or otherwise altering their career paths. This topic will be fully addressed in Chapter 13. But first, we turn to discussion of the stresses faced by physicians during training.

REFERENCES—CHAPTER 11

1. Smye M. Managing the human risks of mergers. In: *Lessons Learned From Mergers & Acquisitions.* Philadelphia, Pa: Right Management Consultants; 1999:42.

2. Tacy B. *Coping with Change.* Niles, Ill: Nightengale-Conant Corp; 1995.

3. Harper-Neeld E. Change awareness (workshop manual). Baton Rouge, La: Shell, Inc; 1995.

4. Rotter JB. Generalized expectancies for internal vs. external control of reinforcement. *Psycholog Monogr.* 1966;80:Whole No. 609.

5. Presson PK, Benassi VA. Locus of control orientation and depression symptomotology: A meta analysis. *J Soc Behav Pers.* 1996;11:201-212.

6. Spector PE. Development of the work locus of control scale. *J Occup Psychol.* 1988;61: 335–340.

7. Spector PE. A consideration of the validity and meaning of self-report measures of job conditions. In Cooper CL, Robertson IT, eds. *International Review of Industrial and Organizational Psychology.* Chichester: Wiley; 1992:123–151.

8. Sotile WM, Sotile MO. *Beat Stress Together: The BEST Way to a Passionate Marriage, Healthy Family, and a Productive Life.* New York, NY: John Wiley & Sons; 1999.

9. Sotile WM, Sotile MO. *The Medical Marriage: Sustaining Healthy Relationships for Physicians and Their Families,* Revised Edition. Chicago, Ill: American Medical Association Press; 2000.

10. Elkind D. *The Hurried Child: Growing Up Too Fast Too Soon.* Reading, Mass: Addison-Wesley; 1981.

11. Lawson E. *The Transformed Self.* Niles, Ill: Nightengale-Conant Corp; 1995.

12. Kilburg RR. *Executive Coaching: Developing Managerial Wisdom in a World of Chaos.* Washington, DC: American Psychological Association, 2000.

13. Prochaska JO, Norcross JC, DiClemente CC. *Changing for Good.* New York, NY: William Morrow & Co; 1994.

14. Amik TL, Ockene JK. The role of social support in the modification of risk factors for cardiovascular disease. In: Shumaker SA, Cajkowski SM, eds. *Social Support and Cardiovascular Disease.* New York, NY: Plenum Press; 1994:259–280.

15. Sotile WM. *Psychosocial Interventions for Cardiopulmonary Patients: A Guide for Health Professionals.* Champaign, Ill: Human Kinetics; 1996.

Understanding and Managing the Stress of Medical Training

"The teaching of good doctoring—of patients, of colleagues, of oneself—should begin in the house staff years."

R Levin[1] (p. 121)

"I can't remember the last time I slept through the night."

A Third-Year Resident

"If I had known medical school would be this brutal, I would have chosen to become an engineer."

A Second-Year Medical Student

"I love this! I'm doing exactly what I've dreamed of doing since I was a kid."

A Fourth-Year Medical Student

"I look back on my years of training with fondness. It was tough, real tough. But my training was top-notch, and the friendships I made during those years have lasted my whole career."

A 58-Year-Old Physician

"A day does not pass without me remembering some aspect of the trauma I went through during my residency. Those were the worst years of my life and I'll never forget or forgive the people who made them that way."

A 42-Year-Old Physician

This chapter systematizes what we know about the stress and coping for physicians-in-training, from medical school through the postgraduate years. We discuss the challenges and pitfalls that come with medical training and interventions that have been tried with students and residents to produce stress-hardy trainees. We systematize information from research with medical students and residents that we have interspersed throughout preceding pages with a wealth of new information on this topic.

It has been argued[2] that undergraduate and postgraduate medical education may not be sufficiently similar to allow comparison. We contend that a discussion combining information about these two populations is useful. Such discussion may help medical students put their current experiences into context and prepare for what is ahead in their education. It may also help residents make sense of their historical, current, and future training experiences. For the sake of clarity, we point out the specific population addressed in referenced works (ie, "students" or "residents"). Otherwise, we use the term "medical trainee" when discussing material that can be applied to both students and residents.

The material in this chapter is also likely to remind experienced physicians of their formative experiences, those that shaped both their professional and personal coping habits. We encourage you to consider the following questions as you proceed: Are you still coping in ways that were shaped by attitudes and behavioral habits formed during your medical training? In which areas of your life are these patterns helpful, and where are they hurting you? Which legacies from your own training are you perpetuating as you deal with the training of others? Is this what you truly want to do?

Self-awareness is empowering. We hope that this look at the issues inherent in the medical training years will promote new levels of insight and empower physicians of all ages to refine their individual coping styles and help colleagues to do the same.

DOES A MEDICAL EDUCATION PUT TRAINEES AT RISK?

The way it *should be:*

"The justification of a university is that it preserves the connection between knowledge and the zest for life. . . . This atmosphere of excitement. . .transforms knowledge. . . . Work. . .is transfused with intellectual and moral vision and thereby turned into a joy, triumphing over its weariness and its pain."[3 (p. 139)]

Few would dispute the nobility of this sentiment, espoused more than 70 years ago. However, debate rages as to whether or not medical training is living up to this standard of excellence. Research on the effects of medical training has brought mixed news.

As of the mid-1990s, studies[4] of medical trainees have failed to demonstrate any definitive links between the stresses of work and health and well-being outcomes. Supporting this contention are investigations like that of Smith et al,[2] whose study of 39 family practice residents and 26 of their spouses via surveys and psychological testing found that residents were handling high levels of stress without major problems. And a recent survey of 1,728 surgical residents[5] reported very low levels of alcohol and substance use and generally positive coping with the extreme stresses of residency. Similarly, Silverman[6] summarized research in this area with the observation that "suicide rates among medical students and residents is not higher than that of age- race- and gender-matched controls in the general population."[6 (p. 105)] Finally, cross-sectional studies have shown that resident couples have marital adjustment scores on standardized tests similar to those of other middle-class and upper–middle-class populations, like young attorneys.[7]

In contrast, a sizable body of research has reported that medical education brings with it a variety of stress-related risks. For example, the aforementioned longitudinal study of 302 medical students[8,9] found that, at follow-up, 33% scored above threshold on a scale that measured symptoms of stress. Coran and Litt[10] surveyed 401 house staff, and of the 70% who responded, 40% of residents indicated that anxiety or depression impaired their performance for a month or more. And Coombs[11] reported that, compared to other graduate-level trainees, resident physicians are 5.5 times more likely to use sleeping pills and stimulants, a pattern that is said to increase the odds of using other drugs like alcohol, psychedelics, and tranquilizers. Finally, Dickstein[12] cautioned that the top and bottom fourth of any medical training class are at greatest risk of abusing alcohol, marijuana, opiates, benzodiazepines, and cocaine.

Concerns have also been expressed that residents may be vulnerable to mismanaging various painful emotional syndromes. Anxiety disorders are said to be the most common group of psychiatric illness among students and residents, just as in the general population.[12] Butterfield[13] noted that depression is probably the most often-cited effect of the stressors of training,[14] but anger is the most often overlooked painful emotion in discussions of resident stress. In fact, three prospective studies of mood changes in resident populations[15-17] found significant increases in anger but not depression. While the debate continues as to whether or not medical training produces symptomatic "casualties," no one proposes that medical training is not stressful.

WHAT STRESSES MEDICAL STUDENTS AND RESIDENTS?

We opened with a quote about the way it *should be*. Here, we offer one perspective on the way it often *is:*

> "Trainees not infrequently see themselves in an adversarial 'we-versus-they' proposition. The 'they' may be patients or senior physicians or hospital administrators who seem distant and uncaring. This adversarial experience probably stems from house-staff disillusionment and alienation within a hospital-training system where they feel powerless and like 'outsiders.' Unlike staff physicians and patients, house officers have a time-limited connection with the hospital."[1 (p. 118)]

Discussion of the stress of medical training is best divided into two areas: the individual developmental course experienced by most medical trainees and the specific stressors that come with the training.

THE DEVELOPMENTAL PERSPECTIVE

Silver[18] noted that "students, while 'eager and enthusiastic' at the time of admission to medical school, became 'cynical,' 'frightened,' 'depressed,' or 'filled with frustration' after spending some time in medical school."[19 (p. 533)] Myers[20] proposed that the stresses of medical school might be compounded by existential questioning that plagues many students from medical families.

> "They may suffer a 'crisis of confidence' or a type of existential career crisis sometime during medical school. Do I really want to be a physician? In my heart am I cut out for medicine? Do I truly enjoy it? Have I indeed given this a lot of thought or am I studying medicine just because my father (mother, or brother, etc) did? I wonder if I'm just looking for acceptance by following in his/her footsteps."[20 (p. 27)]

For most, these self-doubts are transient; for others, they indicate serious underlying personal and family issues that must be addressed.

Residents abruptly switch from student to "physician" and assume high degrees of responsibility for others without commensurate confidence in their ability to do so.[21] It is therefore no wonder that the first postgraduate year has been shown to be, far and away, the most stressful.[22] Aach et al[23] and Girard et al[24] summarized several distinct, chronological stages of resident adjustment as follows:

- *As the first postgraduate year begins, most interns are filled with a positive state of anticipation and excitement.* This is soon replaced by anxieties as self-doubts mount, fueled by recognition of one's limitations. Indeed, the worst stressor for new physicians seems to be caring for people who are dying and concerns about ethical issues.[22] Perhaps this accounts for the observation that intensive-care rotations during the intern year are especially distressing.[22] If the intern is overworked, sleep-deprived, and not supported or encouraged by senior residents or attendings, depression may follow.[23,25] Prospective studies of interns have also documented high levels of anger and hostility during the intern year.[17]

- *The period spanning months three to six of the first year is often a tedious time when activities are stable but uninteresting.* The resident's mood may lift a little, but the tedium proves to be boring. By mid-year, another period of depression is likely as the routine becomes intolerable and work seems endless.

- *By spring, the first-year resident begins to recognize tangible accomplishments and enters a state of success.* Elation and looking forward to assuming the new, more supervisory and academic roles of the second year are typical at the end of year one.[23]

Girard et al[26] observed that, although the second year is less tumultuous and painful than the first, it is still more stressful than the third. A number of researchers[22, 26, 27] have documented that measured levels of stress decrease with the resident's advancing level of training.

Ziegler et al[28] pointed out that the dramas of residency are complicated by the novice physician's attempts to adhere to five commonly held myths:

- Physicians should be all knowing
- Uncertainty is a sign of weakness
- The patient should always come first
- Technical excellence will provide satisfaction
- Patients, not physicians, need support

Such myths contribute to the Rites of Passage perspective of medical training described by Levin[1]: "You need to be a hero to be a physician; if you make it, you join other heroes." Here, stressful medical training is seen to have a "character-building" effect; it provides "conditioning" that prepares the trainee for a grueling life in medicine.

Medical trainees, typically in the early adulthood stage of development, are especially vulnerable to the self-imposed stressors that come from such influences. "House officers frequently over-utilize the character traits of self-reliance and determination that were valuable for acceptance to and completion of medical school."[1 (p. 119)] They learn to see themselves as immune to stress, to ignore it. One unfortunate result for some is the eventual inability to acknowledge fallibility. This leads to a phenomena described as "omnipotent-omniscience" and "I can't say 'no.'" Either can serve to aggravate rather than abate stress.

SPECIFIC STRESSORS

The literature on house staff stress has been criticized as focusing too exclusively on trainee responses to stress and too little on identification of central themes common to all specialties.[1] The following list integrates the themes that have been identified by several reviews of the empirical research in this area.[1,2,13,23,29]

Sleep Deprivation

The long work hours, academic pressures, and, for residents, on-call schedules can lead to both periods of acute sleep loss and chronic sleep deprivation. A recent review of all studies published since 1970 on the subject of the effects of sleep deprivation and fatigue on physicians in training[30] noted a number of research-based concerns in this area:

- Sleep loss correlates with elevations in irritability, hostility, anger, depression, extreme sensitivity to criticism, depersonalization-derealization, and inappropriate affect.

- Sleep loss contributes to elevations of symptoms of depression.

- Short-term tasks requiring manual dexterity and short-term memory are impaired by sleep loss, as is performance on prolonged and repetitive tasks.

- Sleep deprivation when on call affects cognitive processing and emotional state the next day.[31] Specifically, residents have been shown to learn less effectively when tired, presumably due to the fact that fatigue affects storage of information (rather than retrieval).[32]

Working Conditions

Despite concerns about sleep deprivation, several researchers[4,33] have emphasized that no study has yet to demonstrate an association between long hours of work, per se, and health impairment or work performance. *Working conditions*, on the other hand, pose another problem.

In a creative study of United Kingdom residents, Baldwin and colleagues[4] demonstrated how working conditions may actually have differential effects on two variables that affect young physicians: well-being and health. Working long hours one week directly affected residents' *well-being* the next week, as assessed by the General Health Questionnaire (GHQ).[34] Specifically, during the recovery week, exhausted residents showed elevations on measures of somatic symptoms and general social dysfunction. But this was a short-term, transient effect.

On the other hand, the nature of the resident's *work demands*, and not long hours, were found to have a toxic effect on residents' *physical* health. Specifically, over the year studied, the triad of stressors consisting of the number of emergency admissions, the number of deaths, and the amount of time spent fetching (ie, having to go to other wards to fetch things) influenced residents' perceptions of themselves and affected their physical health (measured by elevations on GHQ somatic symptoms). These work demands also correlated with elevations on GHQ measures of anxiety and depression and diminished levels of work performance (measured by self-reported numbers of mistakes).

A Sense of Inadequacy

The relatively high-strain, highly competitive milieu in which they work[35] can contribute to a third, general stressor for medical trainees: a sense of inadequacy. The resident's often ambiguous position—caught some place between being a staff member and an authority figure—combines with work that seems too often filled with difficult patients, difficult patient problems, and information overload.[23] A sense of inadequacy is magnified for anyone who feels forced to cope with problems beyond their competence or experience. When this happens to medical trainees, job satisfaction diminishes.[36]

Loneliness

"A full-time intern or resident is forced to become a part-time spouse, parent, or friend."[1 (p. 118)] Inadequate personal time leaves many residents feeling lonely and isolated from loved ones and dependent on supervisors, other residents, and hospital employees for any sense of support.[37]

Unfortunately, these "supports" often fail to notice or respond to the emotional needs of their peers. Even the perception of low social support has been found to correlate significantly with elevations of resident stress levels.[38] As one resident put it:

> "Everyone in the hospital seems to be living in their own 'silo.' We move through our days doing our jobs in parallel to each other. Everyone is preoccupied with his or her own stress. Then, at the end of another long day, they all seem to go home to their families and I go back up to the floors to finish working up my patients."

Financial Stress

It is not unusual for a young physician to begin his or her career with a six-figure educational debt. For many, the high cost of medical education, coupled with anxiety about the future of the profession and the physician job market, fuels performance pressure. The trainee whose family and/or spouse makes sacrifices to lend financial support may feel a compounding of performance pressure from guilt over the financial burden others are assuming to finance the high cost of his or her medical education.

Academic Trouble

All students and residents enter training having established a track record of academic excellence. But most are ill prepared for the relentlessness and rigor of a medical education. Concerns like those outlined above are magnified in the face of academic struggle. Atypical academic setbacks can lead to a complex of emotions—including disbelief, denial, anguish, sorrow, anger, despair, and/or shame. Some become psychologically devastated.

The student forced to repeat an academic year encounters the further grief of leaving classmates who may have become an important part of his or her support system. The anxiety of joining a new class of strangers mixed with the shock of what may be the first experience with academic "failure" can be paralyzing. The good news is that most students emerge from the repeated year without regret or remorse and with a more positive outlook about their knowledge and education.[20]

Student Abuse

As recently as 1990, Silver and Glicken[39] used the following definition of abuse to analyze responses from 431 medical students at one major medical school.

> "To abuse is to treat in a harmful, injurious, or offensive way; to attack in words; to speak insultingly, harshly, and unjustly to or about a person; to revile;. . .(to engage in) unnecessary or avoidable acts or words of a negative nature inflicted by one person on another person or persons."[39 (p. 527)]

Their report sent shock waves throughout academic medical circles. Forty-six percent of the students surveyed stated they had been abused at some time. Of seniors, 80.6% reported being abused by their senior year. Two-thirds (69.1%) of those abused reported that at least one of the episodes was of "major importance and very upsetting." One-half said the event affected them for a month or longer, and 16.2% said it would "always affect them."

Junior year, when clinical rotations put students in more direct contact with attending and resident physicians, appears to be the year in which students are most likely to report abusive episodes. Fully 23% of the Silver and Glicken[39] sample reported being abused two to five times during their junior year. In contrast, of freshmen, sophomores, and seniors who reported abuse, most reported only one episode of abuse in those years.

In a related study, Sheehan et al[19] surveyed an entire third-year medical school class of 75 students. Their findings confirmed the risks of the third year of training:

■ 85% reported being the target of verbal abuse by residents and interns, clinical faculty, and nurses.

■ 24% reported being threatened with physical harm (by patients and/or interns, residents, or faculty).

■ 47% reported psychological mistreatment, such as being demeaned.

■ 19% reported that other classmates had tried to turn a supervisor against them.

■ Nearly 50% reported that residents or interns and clinical faculty made negative and disparaging remarks about them becoming physicians. Forty percent had heard such comments from nurses.

■ 81% of female medical students reported being targets of sexual harassment. (Fortunately, these same students reported that such harassment was rare in occurrence.)

■ 50% of nonwhite students reported experiencing racial or ethnic slurs.

These surveys suggested that student abuse comes in two predominant "flavors." First is "institutional abuse." Included here are the traditional sources of stress in medical school, such as the heavy work/learning load, anxiety about dissection of cadavers, and so forth. Second is verbal abuse. Here, the perpetrators of student abuse most often are faculty and house staff. One resident described it the *sine quo non* of his training program as "The ABCs: Attack, blame, and criticize."[1 (p. 120)]

Abuse by faculty, residents, and others can alter a young person's capacity to learn and affect the way they cope with the stress of medical training.[39] In the Sheehan et al[19] study, 67% of those abused reported diminished emotional health; 43% reported that the effects of abusive episodes interfered with their family life; and 40% reported negative effects on their physical health.[19]

In addition, many students respond to being abused by questioning their present and future involvement in medicine. Sheehan and associates[19] reported that three-fourths of the abused students stated that they became more cynical about academic life and the medical profession as a result of these episodes. Greater than one-third considered dropping out of medical school, and one-fourth reported they would have chosen a different profession had they know in advance about the extent of mistreatment they would experience.

The factors we have discussed could be termed "the too's:" Too many hours in the hospital; too little sleep; too little time to spend alone with family and friends; too many patients; too little time to study; too much to learn; too little exercise; too many interruptions from beeper calls; too little control over tasks during the working day; too much pressure to not make mistakes; too little money; too much criticism; and too little support. And these are but a few of the stressors that fill the years of medical training.

RELATIONSHIP CHALLENGES FOR MEDICAL TRAINEES

By some estimates, upwards of 25% of students are married when they enter medical school, and 50% to 60% marry before graduation.[20] Coombs and Fawzy's often-cited study of 61 married and unmarried students through 4 years of training found that being married served to buffer students against the stressors of medical school.[40] Other studies[40-44] have clearly demonstrated that marriage and/or strong social contacts can have a buffering effect on the stress perceived by residents.

Strong social support is especially important as well as uniquely challenging for two groups of medical trainees: Those who are gay, lesbian, or bisexual and those who belong to an ethnic minority. We say more about these special groups later. It is true, in general, that the demands of medical training make it difficult to manage the dynamics of personal relationships. Indeed, this may be an understatement. Elsewhere, we have written on this issue:

> "The analogy we suggest when working with couples, one or both of whom is a resident physician, is to think of themselves as if they were 'on point' in a war zone, that is, in the lead position that bears the highest risk and stress of battle formation, and alter their expectations and dealings with each other accordingly. . . .Instead of harboring feelings of resentment toward each other, couples can. . . [recognize] the heroic efforts each one makes to be together during what is often a time of extraordinary stress, challenge, and loneliness."[45 (p. 1180)]

The following 10 factors, which we discuss in detail in the
this section, may pose particular challenges for trainees and
their mates:

- When the Trainee is Lesbian, Gay, or Bisexual (LGB)
- When the Trainee Belongs to a Racial Minority
- When Both Partners are Overworked
- When Feelings of Loneliness and Alienation Accumulate
- When Mates Undergo Different Rates of Adjusting to the
  Training Years
- When Partners Fail to Resolve Tensions and Conflicts
- When Developmental and Maturational Changes Imbalance
  the Relationship
- Extramarital Relationships
- Special Challenges for Dual-Trainee Relationships
- Pregnancy

When the Trainee is Lesbian, Gay, or Bisexual (LGB)

"Medical school and training years typically overlap the young
adult developmental task of finally coming to terms with one's
sexual identity."[12] (p. 175) This can prove to be quite difficult for a
trainee immersed in a medical center culture that may be homophobic. Psychiatrist Michael Myers has written compassionately
on this topic.[20] He cautioned that a homophobic medical education culture can damage the developing sense of self for a gay
student or resident. In addition, such culture can promote illogi-
cal prejudices in heterosexual trainees that may impair their abilities to deliver compassionate support to homosexual colleagues
or compassionate medical care to homosexual patients in the
future. "Slanderous and ignorant remarks by faculty not only
insult the gay and well-informed students but confuse and taint
the poorly informed."[20] (p. 117)

Research indicates that such remarks are far more common
than might be assumed. Townsend and colleagues[46] recently surveyed 320 members of Lesbian, Gay, and Bisexual People in
Medicine, a standing committee of the American Medical Student
Association. One hundred eighty-five students at 92 medical
schools responded. Sixty-two percent (n = 115) of the students

reported that they had been exposed to anti-gay comments during training, and 15% (n = 28) indicated they would not choose to enter the medical field if they were in college today. And recall the aforementioned 1999 survey by Brogan and colleagues[47] in which lesbian physicians reported 4 times more incidents of sexual–orientation-based harassment in medical settings than did their heterosexual colleagues.

Being gay may also directly or indirectly shape a trainee's choice of specialty. Dr Myers pointed out that physicians see themselves as intellectually enlightened and unbigoted, yet "there are members of our profession who would feel nervous about accepting into a pediatric or child psychiatry residency a gay or lesbian applicant. Or reluctant to refer patients to a gay male urologist or lesbian gynecologist."[20 (p. 118)]

Research also supports this contention. In 1998, Ramos and colleagues[48] surveyed 1,949 physicians practicing in New Mexico, questioning them regarding their attitudes toward gay and lesbian trainees and colleagues. Of the 1,044 physicians who responded, only 4.3% stated that they would refuse medical school admission to applicants known to be gay or lesbian. But 10.1% indicated that they were opposed to gay and lesbian physicians seeking residency training in obstetrics and gynecology, and 11.4% indicated that disclosure of homosexual orientation would threaten referrals to gay and lesbian obstetrician–gynecologists. The authors concluded that although physicians' attitudes toward gay and lesbian trainees and colleagues seems to have improved considerably from those reported previously in the literature, gay men and lesbians in medicine continue to face opposition in their medical training and in their pursuit of specialty practice.

Gay and lesbian trainees may even encounter stressful trauma and anxiety about seeking personal medical care. They may fear that being open about their homosexuality will put their academic careers at risk. They may fear that records kept in student health services may not be confidential or that being open with physicians who provide medical care to their institution's trainees may put them at risk of being stigmatized.[20]

Finally, the partners of gay and lesbian trainees may not be accorded the same support as wives and husbands of heterosexual trainees. As a result, they may become increasingly isolated and insular as a couple.

When the Trainee Belongs to a Racial Minority

We reiterate that as recently as 1990, 50% of nonwhite medical students in the United States reported experiencing racial or ethnic slurs.[19] In this sense, Burke and colleagues[49] pointed out that the obstacles facing LGB trainees are similar to those faced by any other minority group within the profession. These obstacles include but are not limited to the following:

"Learning about and understanding a new culture or way of life; speaking and working in a new language; feeling isolated until acquaintances and friends are made; longing for and missing family members and familiar traditions; making dietary, housing, wearing apparel, and other life-style changes; studying and becoming comfortable with disease states and treatment methods specifically North American; preparing for and writing various licensure exams; coming to terms with failure in first attempts at these exams; racial and ethnic discrimination by staff, fellow residents, and patients in the hospital setting; and striking a comfortable personal balance between 'letting go' of some of the old ways and adopting some of the new."[20 (p. 49)]

When Both Partners are Overworked

Landau and associates[42] studied 108 residents and fellows in internal medicine (72% were male, 54% were single, 44% were married, 17% were living with a significant other, 61% of spouses or significant others were either physicians or health care personnel, and only two partners were housewives or not working.) Of those who defined themselves as being in a committed relationship, more than 40% of the respondents reported important problems with their spouse or partner. Of those, 72% believed that these problems were due to the residency, and 61% reported that their spouse or partner agreed with this assessment.

The fact that residency-caused stress may negatively impact one's personal relationship dynamics is not new. The news is that the resident's work stress is not the only job stress that impacts resident marriages; stresses caused by the nonmedical mate's work can also cause relationship strain. How the couple manages this strain will directly affect their perceived levels of support.

When both spouses work, the couple will be stressed by housekeeping responsibilities, child care, and mutual conflicts between professional and family commitments.[42,50,51] Elsewhere[45,52] we cautioned that a nonmedical mate's driven coping style, if mismanaged, can wreak just as much havoc on relationship dynamics as does mismanaged physician stress. Some researchers[7] have suggested that the variable most closely associated with marital adjustment for residents was perceived levels of emotional support given and received *for each other's respective career (including homemaking).*

When Feelings of Loneliness and Alienation Accumulate

One effect of the long work hours required of a trainee is that the student or resident grows isolated and stressed. Not so obvious is the fact that the nonmedical partner now finds him- or herself essentially living alone. This can pose quite a problem for someone who may have made considerable sacrifices, including relocation, in order to facilitate the trainee's medical education. He or she may be left to live in a strange environment without an active support system and with an exhausted, distracted partner. What comes next are various syndromes that may strain the relationship.

The "Medical Student Spouse Syndrome"
Robinson[53] warned of this syndrome, which may arise when students enter the clinical years of training. Unlike the fairly structured first two years of medical school, the clinical years typically bring with them the demand for long absences from home as the student enters the anxiety-laden world of learning to care for real patients at bedside. The mate may refuse to acknowledge that the student is now unavailable and may fail to alter his or her daily routine accordingly. The fantasy that the medical student will show up leads the mate to continue to plan meals or social events. Some spouses may even resort to spending hours outside the medical center, harboring the delusion that the loved one will soon appear.

At first, the medical student may fuel this denial with encouragement that he or she will, indeed, learn to control the work schedule. Complaining may be construed as the partner's attempt to control the overstressed medical student. Eventually, disillusionment and anger set in for each partner.

Loss of Vibrancy

"My partner used to be a lot of fun. Now he/she is just boring." This is a lament that we have heard numerous times when counseling couples during the medical school and residency years. One effect of a trainee's sleep deprivation may be grouchiness, fatigue, and general loss of zest. Even if a "date" is planned, the trainee may fall asleep or be less than enthusiastic due to exhaustion. The quality of time spent together gets worse if the trainee becomes "preoccupied, numb, monosyllabic, irritable, or tyrannical if pushed to engage in domestic or leisure activities."[20 (p. 36)]

Change in Sexual Relations

Fatigue and stress can combine to diminish sex drive for both partners. Myers[20] presented a poignant case vignette describing the plight of the wife of a first-year medical student. She explained her sexual shutdown in these words:

> "I'm the problem. I'm not interested anymore. . . .Let me tell you what's happened to us over the past year. We moved here. . .to start medical school. That wasn't easy because we've left our good friends [back home] and we really haven't made close friends here yet. My mother died six months ago. . .it's still a great loss. . . .I'm not happy with my job here and I may have to make a change. . . . This worry, plus missing my mom, has made me very uptight. I'm eating more and I've gained 15 pounds in 4 months. I hate myself and my body. Bill's out studying at the library every evening during the week, we have supper together then he goes out. When he comes back at ten-thirty or eleven o'clock I'm exhausted and sleepy, that's when he wants to make love. He feels frisky and I feel frumpy. . ."[20 (pp. 9–10)]

When Mates Undergo Different Rates of Adjusting to the Training Years

Disparity may develop between the mates' respective levels of security and enjoyment with this new life. The resident or student may benefit from built-in institutional supports, a professional identity, and, in the case of residents, a secure job, a predictable salary, job structure, and camaraderie with fellow residents. At the same time, the mate may be struggling with feelings of loneliness, failure, and inadequacy about his or her ability to cope with this change.

The relationship is strained when the resident makes suggestions to the mate about how to meet people and to cheer up. These tend to simply lead to more tension, distance, and anger.

The mate's loneliness may be compounded if the physician-in-training wants to socialize with other students or residents and the social times fill with "shop talk." Alternatively, some students and residents prefer to isolate themselves from their peers, leaving the nonphysician spouse without any ready-made points of contact in the new community.

When Partners Fail to Resolve Tensions and Conflicts

As tensions mount, arguments between trainees and their mates tend to follow a familiar pattern. The mate begins to store up feelings of resentment about being shortchanged. The "pedestal effect" may interfere with fruitful discussion of the mate's stresses. Here,

> "the student/resident is treated as a special person because he/she is/will be a physician and therefore considers him or herself above normal responsibilities and respect for his or her partner."[12] (p. 170)

Eventual eruptions leave both parties feeling badly. The trainee feels attacked, blamed, and defensive—"What am I supposed to do? I'm struggling to survive here?" And the mate feels misunderstood and frustrated. Both parties end up feeling guilty, apologetic, and inadequate for not being stronger or more supportive of the other. Things improve and the cycle repeats.[20]

When Developmental and Maturational Changes Imbalance the Relationship

Psychosocial and psychosexual development are fueled by life experiences. For some medical trainees, the pressures, isolation, and abuse that may come their way can stunt psychosocial growth. For others, a true blossoming comes about during the training years. Similar growth and blossoming may happen to one's mate. If not, disequilibrium disrupts the relationship, especially if one mate perceives the other as hampering their growth. Instead of excitement and support from their partner, they may hear "You've changed! You used to be so nice. Now, you are so 'full of yourself!'"

As the training years draw to a close, spousal fears of abandonment are especially likely to be stirred. Everyone has heard a story like this one: "She supported him through medical training and then he left her right at the end of his residency." If left undiscussed and unresolved, these fears can lead to possessiveness, jealousy, arguments, resentment of peers, and general relationship dysfunction at this crucial time.

Extramarital Relationships

Certain scenarios may put medical student/resident marriages at risk of extramarital affairs:[20]

- The spouse may meet and fall in love with someone else because his/her medical trainee wife/husband is totally absorbed in medical study and work.
- The trainee or spouse may feel misunderstood, unloved, or lonely in the relationship.
- Both partners may feel "comfortable," but the relationship may lack depth and intimacy.
- Either partner may feel complacent or bored and look elsewhere for excitement.
- Communication within the relationship may be blocked, resulting in escalating tension that compels both partners to begin to avoid each other.
- Partners in a young marriage with kids at home may react to the hassles of daily life by escaping to a new relationship.
- An individual's personal problems (substance abuse, depression, academic problems, loneliness) may lead to avoidant behaviors, including escaping into a new relationship.

Contemporary researchers[54,55] concerned with the often devastating effect that extramarital affairs have on marriage and family life have emphasized two keys to avoiding the extramarital trap: Keep communication flowing within your relationship and beware of expanding the venues that define relationships with potential extramarital partners.

In this later regard, it is important to be realistic. In today's academic and work settings, learning to work shoulder-to-shoulder with potential suitors is a survival skill. It is only natural that workplace friendships will develop and that, in some instances, "crushes" or otherwise romantic feelings may emerge. Having such feelings is natural; acting on them is optional. To diminish the odds that an extramarital relationships will develop, remember the following risk factors:

■ Beware of moving from a friendship within a confined setting (eg, we see each other in class or at work) to exerting effort to spend time together in a broadening circle of circumstances (eg, you begin going out to lunch together, spending time after work chatting, or traveling together).

■ Do not do things with this person that you would not discuss or do in the presence of your mate.

■ Do not keep secret from your mate your discussions or experiences with the other person.

The stresses outlined thus far take their toll, not only on the relationship but also on both mates. Geurts et al[35] emphasized that failure to receive support from home adds significant stress to the lives of married residents. But let us not forget that no one lives in a vacuum. The trainee's mate, too, is impacted by the stresses that come with a medical education. Underscoring this point is research by Smith et al,[2] who reported that, compared to their resident mates, nonmedical mates evidenced more distress on standard psychological measures than did the residents themselves. This finding prompted the authors to conclude that,

> "Since spouses feel they have to carry more than their share of family responsibilities when their partner is a resident, perhaps educators should focus more attention on reducing stress among spouses as a way to reduce stress for residents."[(p. 403)]

Special Challenges for Dual-Trainee Relationships

Students or residents who are dating or married to other medical trainees in the same institution face a special set of pros and cons. A positive comes in the form of mutual support and familiarity with the stressors of training. Dual trainees often remind us of how individuals in dual-physician marriages tend to benefit from their shared passion for medicine and their joint tolerance of the long hours required by "the angry mistress, medicine."

On the "con" side, dual-trainee couples may find that they tire of feeling like they live in a goldfish bowl. "There is a sense that the whole class is observing and tracking their every move."[20 (p. 22)] Still others find that academic competition with their mate—sometimes fueled by friends and family who serve as their "audience"—may generate relationship tensions.

Any dual-career couple is vulnerable to the stresses that come with having to make decisions about whose career will take priority when deciding such issues as whether or not to relocate in order to pursue one partner's career advancement. We have spent much of our career counseling such couples, and, elsewhere, we have written extensively on these experiences.[50,51]

It is our opinion that relationship dynamics are especially stressful for dual-trainee couples. This complexity tends to peak at the time of applying for and matching for residencies. How the couple determines whose residency choice will take priority can have profound effects on the immediate and long-range future of the relationship. Some couples simply end their relationship in order to allow each partner to finish their educational quest. Others compromise. Each settles for a "less-than-best" residency placement. Most strike some form of "bargain" that involves one partner deferring to the other's first choice of residency with the promise that, at some point in the future, the compromising partner will have the favor of deference to his or her career needs returned.

Pregnancy

Since 1970, the number of women physicians has quadrupled, and it has been estimated that by 2010 approximately 30% of practicing physicians in the United States and an even greater percentage of medical trainees will be women.[56]

The special challenges faced by women during medical training have been well documented. These include but are not limited to gender-based discrimination, sexual harassment, and a relative lack of female medical role models.[57,58]

Our experiences as speakers to gatherings of medical trainees have afforded us numerous anecdotal reports of the special challenges faced by women today. Single female trainees complain that it is difficult to establish and/or maintain dating relationships.

Two hurdles they frequently mention are lack of time and the intimidation factor.

One woman explained the first of these in this way:

> "Compared to the single guy students, it seems to be tougher for us. I'll meet a guy, have a nice date or two, but then I 'disappear' for weeks on end. These clinical rotations take up more time than people can imagine. Guys who aren't in medical school seem to either not believe me when I tell them 'Sorry, I'd like to go out with you again, but I'm tied-up for the foreseeable future.' Or, they just aren't willing to wait. I guess it's not part of the guy role to wait. My fellow male medical students don't seem to have the same difficulty. They have the same time constraints, but the women they date seem to be more tolerant of their schedules; more willing to wait long periods between dates."

Other women report that their status as a medical trainee seems to intimidate potential suitors.

> "I just don't get it," one woman stated. "Why does the fact that I'm a physician have to be such an issue? These days, compared to many during the past 4 years, I actually have a little more time available to socialize. But as soon as a new acquaintance finds out I'm a resident, they seem to get nervous. Like I'm too smart or something. More people have a 'physician mystique' than you'd think. And it's messing up my love life!"

Perhaps this combination of factors contributes to the observation that, although the transition from medical school to residency seems to improve quality of life for males, not so for females. Hendrie et al[27] studied 634 medical students and 227 house staff and found that, while the proportion of men reporting anxiety and depressive symptoms declined between medical school (33%) and residency (10%), no such decline occurred with women (medical students 42%, residents 37%).

For many women trainees, their most bittersweet challenges come when they get pregnant. Approximately two-thirds of all practicing women physicians have children. Nearly 50% of these women gave birth during residency, and 13% had their first child during fellowship.[59] Approximately one quarter of all women physicians with children had more than one child during residency,[60] and 63% of pregnancies during graduate medical training are planned.[61]

In a thoughtful discussion, Ducker[58] argued that studies of role conflict among female physicians suffer from the error of assuming that this is a homogenous group. Overall, women physicians report high levels of satisfaction with their work/ home balance. However, the experiences of a sizable subset of women mothers is more complicated. On the one hand, some women report that multiple role involvement brings new privileges that can reduce the cost of added roles and even lead to rewards.[58] For others physicians, pregnancy and motherhood create soul-splitting dilemmas. In a nutshell, Ducker argues that the greater their commitment to their professional life, the greater the role strain experienced by physician mothers. Research suggests that, post-training, most physician mothers tend to claim that they place a higher priority on family than on their careers. For example, in Sells' study of female pediatricians,[62] 73% stated that they put family first, while 14% stated they put career first, and 13% gave both equal importance.

While it may be possible for a woman who has completed her medical training to clearly prioritize family over career, it is difficult to do so during the intense training years. For decades, women physicians have indicated that they were made to feel embarrassed and ashamed of getting pregnant during training; that their "commitment to the profession" was questioned by their decision to become or to remain pregnant; and that they encountered hostility from their superiors and/or colleagues.[60] As recently as 1989, only 47.8% of 366 training hospitals surveyed granted formal maternity leave.[63] This perhaps contributes to the rather high abortion rate that has been reported among residents in some specialties. A National Institutes of Health study of 4,412 women residents reported an 8.7% abortion rate across all specialties. Surgical residents reported the highest abortion rate (22.3%), while pathology and radiology were the lowest at 1.9% and 2.3%, respectively.[64] A study of plastic surgery residents[65] found an abortion rate of 26%.

Given the age of medical trainees, it is clear that they and their faculty must adopt realistic strategies for dealing with pregnancy during the training years. Both male and female residents must accept that it is probable that, directly or indirectly, their course of training is likely to be impacted by someone's pregnancy—if not their own, then that of a colleague. Faculty have to develop both formal and informal support systems for pregnant residents and institutional policies regarding maternity leave, coverage, and so forth. We propose that the following five factors be considered by all concerned when evaluating this issue.

Be Aware of the Group Dynamics That May Come With a Resident's Pregnancy

A qualitative study of a small group of psychiatry residents who became pregnant during training[66] highlighted many of the dynamics we have observed when we have counseled pregnant residents. The authors reported that nonpregnant resident colleagues viewed the pregnant residents as being "selfish" or "entitled" and complained that the pregnant women had been treated specially by the residency administration. Nonpregnant residents also expressed resentment over the increased coverage demands placed on them when a colleague left for maternity leave. Interestingly, resentment was also expressed over the observation that the quality of interaction among pregnant and nonpregnant residents deteriorated. Here, the nonpregnant residents complained that they tired of ongoing talk of parenting issues and missed interaction around patient and education issues.

The pregnant residents in this study[66] admitted that, during their pregnancies, they had felt distracted from work, both emotionally and physically, particularly later in pregnancy. They also complained that, although they found a nonpregnant woman resident colleague to be "distant but supportive," the responses of all the men were uniformly negative, including anger, resentment, and sarcasm.

Anger and hostility toward pregnant residents has been reported in various specialties.[60] It also has been posed that the anger and resentment that pregnant residents perceive in others may be influenced by projection of their own ambivalence about being pregnant at this time in their career.[66,67]

Pregnant residents generally report that they perceive more support from faculty than they do from peers. Eskenazi and Weston[65] proposed that this may be due to miscommunication between the pregnant resident and her resident colleagues. In truth, all residents benefit from a show of understanding of the unique pressures they experience. The pregnant woman, focused as she may be on personal preoccupation with her pregnancy, may ignore the work implications her pregnancy might pose for her colleagues. The colleagues, on the other hand, may mistakenly interpret that the resident is not committed to her career. With the resident feeling devalued and the colleagues feeling abandoned, failure to discuss this process fuels tension.

Know the "Typical" Time-Off Scenario

Pregnant residents continue to work up until a mean of 12 days prior to delivery, with 52% working up until the day before or the day of delivery.[65,68,69] In 1991, the Women in Medicine Advisory Panel surveyed residency program directors.[56] Approximately 75% of the 1,200 directors who responded said their programs have standard maternity leave policies. Thirty-eight percent allowed more than 6 weeks of leave, 37% allowed between 4 and 6 weeks, and 24% allowed fewer than 4 weeks.[56] In Canada, paid maternity leave for all workers, including medical residents, is 17 to 20 weeks.[70] The vast majority of women residents return from pregnancy leave to work full time.[71]

The length of pregnancy leave taken by female residents has been found to be significantly less than that of the working spouses of their male colleagues.[72]

Residents are well advised to investigate their specialty's regulations governing certification before taking extended leaves, regardless of the leave allowance of their residency program.[73] In 1987, the typical specialty board allowed 4 to 6 weeks of leave, but some boards only allowed as little as 2 weeks leave per year.[56]

Consider These Questions

As recently as 1990, it was the case that in two-thirds of academic and private departments in certain specialties (eg, radiology),[74] women were informed of the pregnancy and maternity leave policy only on request.

"This puts the prospective employee or residency candidate in the uncomfortable position of having to bring up the subject and intensifies the fear that by raising the question, she will be at a disadvantage."[74] (p. 328)

To evaluate a residencies maternity leave policies, consider these questions:[60,68,75]

- Is leave allowed for adoptions and paternity?
- What is the duration of sick leave allowed before and after delivery?
- Is leave paid or unpaid?
- Is leave designed to supplant vacation?
- Can leave be extended by adding accrued vacation time?
- Is provision made for continuation of insurance benefits?

- Is it permissible to return to work on a part-time basis for the first few weeks after maternity leave?
- Can sick leave and vacation time be accrued from year to year or used in advance?
- Will makeup time be paid and how will it be reimbursed?
- Does the residency program director have a record of being supportive of pregnant residents?

Carefully Consider the Option of Postponing Pregnancy
Fully 70% of the female physicians in Sinal's 1988 national survey[57] advised that the best time to become pregnant was "after completion of residency." Forty-three percent of these women spoke from experience: They had become pregnant during internship and residency. In addition, the "best advice" offered by many department chairs polled was simple: "postponement of pregnancy."[65] Of course, this option must be weighed against the fact that postponement carries increased risk of complications, increased severity of complications, and increased incidence of infertility.[76]

Learn the Characteristics of Pregnancy-Friendly Residencies
Eskenazi and Weston[65] outlined nine suggestions to physician leaders who shape pregnancy policies. Collectively, these suggestions describe what would be a very pregnancy-friendly residency program.

- Institute a policy that encourages women to inform their department chair(s) of their pregnancy by the beginning of the second trimester in order to plan rotations equitably.
- Formulate specific maternity leave policies that incorporate resident input.
- Offer around-the-clock childcare for all hospital employees.
- Encourage more women role models who juggle medical careers and family responsibilities.
- Build in rotations without night call or buffers of elective time or a research year.
- Explore job-sharing options if feasible.
- Reward those residents who are willing to take extra night call.
- Allow call exchange so pregnant residents can make up call prior to delivery.

■ Allow open discourse regarding the timing of pregnancy and family issues.

WHAT CAN BE DONE TO HELP MEDICAL TRAINEES TO COPE?

A bit of good news for hard-working medical trainees comes from Meijman's effort-recovery model.[77] This model proposes that dealing with high work load and developing mental or emotional strains during the workday is not necessarily unhealthy; the key is to recover sufficiently during the nonworking hours.

The medical training years are so filled with high-demand work stresses that students and residents cannot afford to be lax about practicing appropriate self-care habits. Research with resident populations has documented the importance of simple stress management strategies like making time for moderate amounts of physical exercise,[42] periodically escaping from the rigors of work,[24] and taking advantage of available times to catch up on sleep.[78] Simply making time for frequent, brief visits with friends and relatives has been found to attenuate the negative effects of high levels of work stress for residents.[42]

Throughout this book, trainees will find guidelines for honing their coping skills. In the remainder of this chapter, we elucidate what training institutions and physician leaders can do to bolster trainee coping skills and provide them with adequate support systems.

Identify the At-Risk Trainee

One key to promoting stress-hardy trainees is the early detection, diagnosis, and treatment of individuals who are at risk of poor adaptation to new roles and responsibilities.[6] Some authors[79] have recommend that, based on the trainee stress research literature, some trainees must be recognized as being at risk. At-risk groups include those just entering or about to leave training; unmarried residents; female residents; and residents with a minority religious, cultural, or racial background. In addition, at risk are those who begin their medical careers with traits of insecurity, low self-esteem, dependency, social anxieties, proneness to depression, tendency to obsessively worry, low self-confidence, passivity, and social withdrawal.[80]

T a b l e   12-1

Work–Home Characteristics of At-Risk Residents

Work Characteristics	Home Characteristics
An unfavorable work time schedule	Part of a dual-career couple
High workload	Partner who works overtime frequently
High mental workload	Have children
Lack of job autonomy	Trouble arranging flexible child care
High dependency on the superior	Experience little support from home

Source: Geurts S, Rutte C, Peeters M. Antecedents and consequences of work-home interference among medical residents. *Soc Sci Med.* 1999;48:1135–1148.

As was previously mentioned (see Chapter 1), particular concerns have been expressed that medical students and residents who are highly self-critical tend to manifest high levels of later-career stress and to experience difficulties in their relationships with senior colleagues.[8] Individuals who are in the top fourth and those in the bottom fourth of any medical training class are at greatest risk of adjustment problems like substance abuse.[12] In our experience, mismanaged perfectionism is one factor that may underlie this observation. Perfectionism can cause problems of two distinct sorts. On the one hand, some trainees channel their perfectionistic tendencies into overachievement quests that leave them distressed and prone to inappropriate self-management. Others mismanage their perfectionistic tendencies, leaving them paralyzed and compromised in their ability to perform adaptively. Both syndromes signal the need for interventions that teach trainees to shape realistic, adaptive attitudes and constructive coping skills.

Also at risk of struggling are those trainees suffering high job stress and low social support.[81] Trainees who struggle with work–home interference have been found to be at particular risk. Here, difficulties may be bi-directional: The individual may experience pressures within the work domain that are incompatible with role demands within the family[35] or family demands may interfere with work performance.[82] In either case, measures of trainee distress elevate and health indicators diminish.[35]

Table 12-1 summarizes the characteristics of those residents at risk of experiencing work–home interference.[35]

While we underscore the importance of early detection of psychosocial struggles and intervention with residents, we also offer two points of caution in this regard. First, avoid the mistake of interpreting normal reactions to stress as symptoms of pathology.[1] Remember, as a group, medical trainees are a happy and hardy lot. Most adjustment struggles will prove to be transient, especially if the trainee is treated with respect and afforded appropriate support.

Second, be aware that the task of identifying trainees who are struggling may be more difficult than it appears. In a creative study, Purdy et al[83] assessed whether residency directors and psychologist faculty could accurately predict the presence and degree of burnout among their family practice residents. Residency directors were more accurate than psychologist faculty in identifying which residents saw themselves as most burned out, but directors significantly underestimated the level of burnout, where psychologists did not. Most interesting was the finding that neither medical director nor behavioral faculty were able to accurately identify which residents saw themselves as burned out in the first year. Both faculty groups made accurate identifications of second-year residents, and only the medical directors accurately rated burnout in third-year residents. The authors speculated that the underestimation of burnout in first-year residents may be contributed to by a tendency of residency directors, having themselves endured medical training, to minimize the significance of signs of burnout that they see.

Manage Work Hours

Since the mid 1980s, medical educators worldwide have grappled with the question of how stress might be reduced without compromising the goals of good training.[1 (p. 120)]

In the United States, a 1987 Ad Hoc Advisory Committee on Emergency Services examined working conditions and supervision of residents in teaching hospitals. This endeavor came about in response to public outcry over the death in 1984 of a young woman in a New York City hospital that was attributed to medical mistakes made by a sleep-deprived resident. The committee concluded that the current system was having an adverse effect on the personal lives and attitudes of residents toward themselves and their patients. They also found evidence of high levels of resident anger, cynicism toward patients, depression, suicidal ideation, substance abuse, and interference with their family lives.[84] The committee made the following recommendations:[85]

- Interns, residents, and attending physicians should work no more than 12 consecutive hours in hospitals with more than 15,000 emergency department visits.
- Interns and residents should not work more than an average of 80 hours a week over a 4-week period.
- Interns and residents should not be scheduled to work for more than 24 consecutive hours, to be separated by no fewer than 8 nonworking hours and with at least one 24-hour period of nonworking time each week.
- Provisions should be made for on-site, in-person supervision of trainees.

A similar initiative has been ongoing in Britain since the early 1990s. Termed "The New Deal,"[86] this set of guidelines mandated that British physicians not work more than 72 hours a week.

The results of such initiatives have been quite mixed. On the one hand, the reduced total working hours and the removal of inappropriate duties have lessened residents' sense of being overwhelmed.[87] In addition, there is some evidence that these changes have improved the quality of the medical care delivered by residents. When changes in their work hours have resulted in increased sleep regularity, residents have been found to make fewer medication errors, request fewer laboratory tests, and effectively treat patients with shorter lengths of hospital stay.[78]

On the other hand, because work hours have lessened but work demands have not, British physicians have complained of increased work intensity. In addition, British residents have had to adjust to ongoing changes in their work patterns. As more and more physician tasks are taken on by nurses, phlebotomists, and ward clerks, confusion between nursing and phlebotomists' roles and those of resident physicians has increased resident stress levels.[87] This later finding is related to the documented fact that understanding one's task and role clarity increases job satisfaction and diminishes stress among senior house officers.[88]

Finally, while the New Deal led to welcomed relief from the stress of overwork, young physicians and their supervisors have expressed concern that they may not be gaining adequate hands-on supervised medical experience.[21]

It is generally accepted that resident stress levels are, indeed, lessened by certain institutional policies that lighten their workload. These include reduced amounts of night call[89] and monitoring

of work schedules, patient caseloads, and on-call rotations to minimize unnecessary and harmful emotional and physical fatigue.[1]
However, beyond a point of rather modest changes in the work
demands, it appears that equally or more important are interventions and attitudes among training institutions and their faculty
that recognize and help to ameliorate resident stressors. These
include providing mentors, peer support, and a menu of support
services, all geared toward teaching the skills needed to deal with
the hospital environment. These skills include the ability to communicate, to organize one's efforts, to engage in teamwork, and to
achieve a reasonable work-family balance.[1,90]

Provide Mentors and Other Means of Curbing Trainee Abuse

Since the mid 1980s, visionary physicians[91-93] have touted the
advisability of nonadversarial collegiality. The importance of
heeding this call cannot be overemphasized and is supported by
research on physician well-being. When managed appropriately,
frequent contact with faculty physicians serves as a major compo-
nent of housestaff satisfaction.[92] But a wealth of contemporary
researchers[35,94,95] have documented that one of the most toxic stressors for residents is a problematic relationship with a superior.
The worse the relationship, the more psychosomatic health complaints reported by the residents and the more the residents had
cynical and distant attitudes towards patients and colleagues.[35]

Levinson et al[96] emphasized that mentors should be guides or
hosts who influence the trainee's intellectual, personal, and professional growth. "Successful mentoring in medicine requires educators and trainees to acknowledge their mutual stresses, needs,
and ambitions."[1 (p. 20)] Levinson also emphasized that the mentoring
relationship can be harmful if, rather than offering valuable moral
and personal support, the mentor relationship fills with unhealthy
competition between the mentor and junior colleague.

It is important to think systematically about this issue of the
trainee/superior relationship. Levin[1] cautioned that

"one should not be quick to blame medical educators, as changes in hospital
training programs and faculty teaching practices over the past 30 years have
undermined consistent and optimal teacher–trainee relationships. The growth of
specialties, the evolution of the teaching hospital in large academic medical

centers, and the emphasis on multiple training sites for diversity of experience and income for the department may all militate against the development of relationships conducive to optimal training."[1] [(p. 119)]

Levin[1] also outlined various factors that might promote ineffective mentoring in today's medical setting:

- Competition for positions and patients may be intense.
- Male physicians may have inadequate experience in mentoring women.
- Senior physicians may become insecure and defensive when faced with ever-changing biotechnical advances.
- Medical educators may use intellectual one-upmanship to maintain authority in a field where their trainees are often closer to advances in knowledge.

Silver and Glicken[39] offered astute observations about the systemic aspects of resident/student abuse. Residents may feel that students' performance will reflect directly or indirectly on the residents and may feel forced to participate in education of students even though they might not have the time, desire, or ability to carry out this function.

Finally, medical students' own recommendations for the prevention and management of abuse are worth noting:[39]

- Educate faculty, residents, and staff as to the rights of students. Emphasize that the areas of student abuse and sexual harassment share an interesting distinguishing feature: Perceptions take priority over intentions.
- Appoint a grievance committee or a group of ombudsmen to investigate complaints of abuse.
- Establish a mechanism to discipline abusers.
- Reward faculty who are particularly considerate and understanding of students.
- Initiate institutional reform to decrease the possibility of abuse taking place.
- Offer counseling to all parties involved with abusive episodes.
- Take measures to be fair to all sides in a reported episode of abuse. Protect those who may be unfairly accused of abusive behavior.

Recognize That LGB and Minority Trainees Have Special Needs for Support

Surveys of LGB trainees have underscored the importance of providing them with faculty liaisons and support groups.[46,97] Medical training should include experiences that heighten awareness of the following issues:

- The special challenges faced by LGB trainees[98–100]
- Issues that affect LGB patient care[46,97]
- The need for training programs to be proactive in acknowledging and supporting diversity of sexual orientation[97]
- How sexual orientation influences health care delivery[101]

Of course, insisting that policies censuring discrimination based on sexual orientation or ethnicity be strictly adhered to is a must in today's training environment.[97] But it is also important that medical leaders role-model tolerance and compassion for diverse populations of colleagues and patients.

Given the large population of foreign-born medical trainees currently enrolled in American institutions, it is also important to recognize their special needs for support. The fact that foreign students may fear disclosing any problems in an unfamiliar culture and institution can significantly complicate their management of stress-related concerns. A minority trainee in need of counseling is likely to encounter the additional hurdle of finding a health care provider who is both versed and respectful of their cultural mores. The importance of finding counseling and medical services that are respectful of one's ethnicity has been well documented.[102]

Promote Peer Support

It is no surprise that research has documented that social support[81] and, specifically, peer group cohesion[103] attenuates the effects of trainee stress. Simply put, as levels of support rise, levels of measured stress diminish. A number of creative efforts at reducing trainee stress by promoting social support and group cohesion have been reported in the literature. Two representative examples are described below.

Mushin et al[104] detailed a comprehensive, 12-session support program offered at the Baylor College of Medicine, Department of Medicine. During their monthly support group meetings, first-

T A B L E   12-2

Support Group Curriculum

Topic	Strategies
Time management	Divide the group according to rotations; have senior residents offer helpful "shortcuts" in daily functions and other organizational tips
Interactions with nurses	Case simulation of potential conflicts with nurses
Interactions with difficult patients	Discussion and handouts regarding code status Group discussion of ethical issues Case presentations
Dealing with difficult families	Case simulation; discuss families and family dynamics
Management of medical mistakes	Senior residents discuss medical mistakes they have made and situations in which residents should exercise extra caution
Interaction with senior staff	Cases of difficult interactions between senior residents and attending physicians taking into consideration various personality types
Handling grief	Strategies for recognizing and assisting self, patients, and families with grief
Quality control circle	Planned group problem solving and short- and long-term efficiency flows in system
Patient–physician interaction	Group meetings with special patient panel to discuss physician–patient relationship issues
Strategies for senior residents	Case simulations of problems senior residents encounter; panel discussions; discussion of leadership strategies

Source: Mushin IC, Matteson MT, Lynch EC. Developing a resident assistance program: Beyond the support group model. *Arch Intern Med.* 1993;153:729–733. Used with permission.

year residents are presented with typical, difficult situations they are likely to encounter, and, with the guidance of senior residents who serve as group leaders, strategies are developed. The list of topics and recommended strategies included in the Mushin et al[104] intervention are outlined in Table 12-2. This program demonstrates how a support group can provide far more than a series of gripe sessions; this program promotes a range of coping skills that can serve residents in a wide spectrum of situations.

Matthews et al[105] reported on a similar program for addressing the emotional needs of house staff members in internal medicine. Offered at the University of Connecticut Affiliated Hospitals, this program utilizes three full-day sessions conducted immediately prior to the start of internship and five half-day sessions spaced equally at 6-week intervals.

Offer a Menu of Support Services

A survey of 576 residencies across six specialties in 1988–1989 found that despite recent attention to residents' working hours and conditions, many programs in many specialties did not yet offer a variety of effective support services for residents during training.[106] This is unfortunate, given that support groups and other supportive services have been identified by residents to be both desirable[107] and effective.[2] Such programs appear to be especially effective in combating feelings of isolation and affording opportunity to ventilate negative feelings and receive support from one's peers. They may also prevent impairment among some residents.[106]

Many options are available for providing medical trainees support. Kahn and Addison[106] and Smith et al[2] outlined the following options.

- Confidential professional counseling with counselors available within the residency at reduced or no fee, or benefits supplied by the residency or hospital for counseling (Note: 30% of pediatric and anesthesiology residents and 60% of psychiatry residents said they would use confidential individual psychotherapy if it were available.[107])
- Ongoing support groups for residents
- Support groups for significant others or spouses and for couples
- Balint-type seminars that focus on exploring the dynamics of troubling physician–patient relationships
- Seminars or speakers dealing with emotionally charged medical issues (for example, the dying patient)
- Seminars or speakers dealing with the stresses and conflicts of being a physician

- Seminars or speakers that teach management and communication skills
- Financial advisors to help residents deal with financial concerns
- Formal "gripe sessions" that provide an avenue for voicing complaints and requests for program change
- Resident participation on committees that deal with residency curriculum decision making
- Part-time residency option
- Alternative residency scheduling that involves time off without lengthening the duration of the residency (eg, residency-sponsored "mental health" days, post-call time off)
- Social activities planned and sponsored by the residency
- Retreats that afford all residents opportunities to get away from the program together, with coverage provided by the program
- Orientation—a week- or month-long program for new residents with limited patient care responsibilities
- Child care services such as day care or baby-sitting services sponsored by the residency program or hospital

Kahn and Addison[106] concluded in their review of support services currently available to medical residents that the most frequently offered types of support services are residency-sponsored social activities, professional counselors on staff, and seminars and/or speakers dealing with emotionally charged medical issues. Compared to the 1980s, more residencies in the 1990s offered seminars and speakers dealing with stress and conflicts of being a physician. This, perhaps, reflects increased concern for and attention to residents' well-being. Family practice programs were found to be more likely to offer support groups and various seminar-type experiences.[106] And a survey of family practice residents and their spouses conducted by Smith et al[2] found that a residents' support group and relaxation therapy were the top two choices, while counseling for individuals and/or couples was their third preference.

The following list calls attention to several outstanding support programs that have been reported in the literature:

- The University Medical Center, University of Arizona, Tucson offers an 8-week meditation-based stress reduction intervention with premedical and medical students.[108]
- The University of Wisconsin (Madison) Department of Pediatrics holds a faculty-house staff retreat every 2 years that fosters group communication to reduce stress.[109]
- Various specialties offer leadership conferences for chief residents (eg family practice residents).[110]
- Half-day workshops that teach management of the stress of medical practice have been recommended.[111]
- The University of Louisville Medical Student Health Promotion and Prevention Program is made available to all entering medical students and their significant others. This program is held 4 days before the mandatory orientation day. Presentations by faculty and "health tutors" regarding physical and emotional health are combined with opportunities to meet other students and residents and to get to know about the school and facilities, support services, and support persons available. This program also makes available to all faculty at department meetings ongoing presentations regarding sexual harassment and medical student abuse.[12]

A special publication by the Committee for the Association of Program Directors in Internal Medicine[23] offered a menu of options for providing various forms of support to medical trainees and their families. A summary of these recommendations is presented in Table 12-3.

We close this discussion with two caveats. First, Kaplan and Marshall[112] recommended that program directors and others responsible for support programs in residency training be aware of and anticipate resistance to support measures. Based on a small study of resident attitudes toward support services and those who access them, the authors recommended that some residents may need help to learn to be comfortable seeking help and to respect help-seeking in others. They also recommended that faculty arrange for support group members to cross-cover for one another, in order to avoid forcing other peers to make sacrifices for those seeking support.

T A B L E   12-3

Various Forms of Support for Medical Trainees

Type of Stress	Solutions
Family	Social activities, family group meetings, maternity and paternity policies
Financial	Formal instructions about debts, budgets, and financial planning; defined program policies on moonlighting
Isolation; problems of relocating	Orientation, informational gripe sessions, retreats with faculty, encourage peer interaction outside the patient care arena, big brother and sister programs, social activities, provide chamber of commerce materials
Lack of leisure time	Formal instruction on time management, mandated and personal days off, encourage athletics and outside interests
Psychosocial problems	Established policies for early identification of impairment, counseling, change of schedule, leave of absence if required; inform residents at orientation of policies and availability of professional assistance; group sessions
Inadequate coping skills	Formal instruction, individual counseling

Source: Aach RD, Cooney TG, Girard DE, et al. Stress and impairment during residency training: Strategies for reduction, identification, and management. *Ann Intern Med.* 1988; July 15:154–161.

CONCLUSIONS

Medical training is and will continue to be stressful. Eliminating trainee stress is not the goal; building resilient trainees is. The habits and values trainees develop for coping with stress will, like their clinical skills, extend into their post-training careers and affect their resilience.[1] We hope that our overview of this complex issue will serve to stimulate further discussion and research in this area.

In closing, the findings of Girard and colleagues[24] are worth noting. These researches reported that, when asked what would help ameliorate the stress of training, senior residents identified only changes that allowed for their "escape" from the hospital as potentially helpful. They did not identify improved social outlets, relationships with faculty, or even improved didactic sessions as particularly useful, nor the availability of counseling services.

This finding underscores the importance of promoting both the opportunities and the skills trainees need in order to remain stress hardy. Policies that govern vacation time, levels of administrative help, and amounts of night call must be monitored. At the same time, trainees must be taught the value of creating and taking advantage of regular, small "recesses" from work that allow them to rest, relax, and rejuvenate their energies.

REFERENCES—CHAPTER 12

1. Levin R. Beyond "The men of steel": The origins and significance of house staff training stress. *Gen Hosp Psychiatry.* 1988;10:114–121.

2. Smith MF, Andrasik F, Quinn SJ. Stressors and psychological symptoms of family practice residents and spouses. *J Med Educ.* 1988; 63:397–405.

3. Whitehead AN. Universities and their function. In: *The Aims of Education.* London, England: Ernest Benn Ltd; 1932:138–139.

4. Baldwin PJ, Dodd M, Wrate RW. Young doctors' health–1. How do working conditions affect attitudes, health and performance? *Soc Sci Med.* 1997;45:35–40.

5. Bunch WH, Dvonch VM, Storr CL, Baldwin DC, Hughes PH. The stresses of the surgical residency. *J Surg Res.* 1992;53:268–271.

6. Silverman MM. Physicians and suicide. In: Goldman LS, Myers M, Dickstein LJ, eds. *The Handbook of Physician Health.* Chicago, Ill: American Medical Association; 2000:95–117.

7. Spendlove DC, Reed B, Whitman N, Slattery ML, French TK, Horwood K. Marital adjustment among housestaff and new attorneys. *Acad Med.* 1990;65(9):599–603.

8. Firth-Cozens J. Predicting stress in general practitioners: 10 year follow-up postal survey. *BMJ.* 1997;315:34–35.

9. Firth-Cozens, J. Individual and organisational predictors of depression in general practitioners. *Brit J Gen Prac.* 1998;1647–1651.

10. Coran LM, Litt IF. Housestaff well-being. *West J Med.* 1988;148:97–101.

11. Coombs RH. *Drug-Impaired Professionals.* Cambridge, Mass: Harvard University Press; 1997.

12. Dickstein LJ. Medical students and residents: Issues and needs. In: Goldman LS, Myers M, Dickstein LJ, eds. *The Handbook of Physician Health. Chicago,* Ill: American Medical Association; 2000:161–179.

13. Butterfield PS. The stress of residency: A review of the literature. *Arch Intern Med.* 1988;148:1428–1435.

14. Reuben DB. Depressive symptoms in medical house officers: Effects of level of training and work rotation. *Arch Intern Med.* 1985;145:286–288.

15. Ford CV, Wentz DK. The internship year: A study of sleep, mood states, and psychophysiologic parameters. *South Med J.* 1984;77:1435–1442.

16. Gordon GH, Hubbell FA, Wyle FA, et al. Stress during internship. *J Gen Intern Med.* 1986;1:228–231.

17. Uliana RL, Hubbell FA, Wyle FA, et al. Mood changes during the internship. *J Med Educ.* 1984;59:119–123.

18. Silver HK. Medical students and medical school. *JAMA.* 1982; 247:309–310.

19. Sheehan A, Sheehan DV, White K, Leibowitz A, Baldwin DC. Pilot study of medical student 'abuse." Student perceptions of mistreatment and misconduct in medical school. *JAMA.* 1990;263:533–537.

20. Myers MF. *Doctors' Marriages: A Look at the Problems and Their Solutions.* New York, NY: Plenum; 1988.

21. Moss F, Paice E. Getting things right for the doctor in training. In: Firth-Cozens J, Payne R, eds. *Stress in Health Professionals: Psychological and Organisational Causes and Interventions.* New York, NY: John Wiley & Sons; 1999:203–218.

22. Schwartz AJ, Black ER, Goldstein MG, Jozefowicz RF, Emmings FG. Levels and causes of stress among residents. *J Med Educ.* 1987;62:744–753.

23. Aach RD, Cooney TG, Girard DE, et al. Stress and impairment during residency training: Strategies for reduction, identification, and management. *Ann Intern Med.* 1988;5:154–161.

24. Girard DE, Hickam DH, Gordon GH, Robison RO. A prospective study of internal medicine residents' emotions and attitudes throughout their training. *Acad Med.* 1991;66:111–114.

25. Firth-Cozens J, Greenhalgh J. Doctors' perceptions of the links between stress and lowered clinical care. *Soc Sci Med.* 1997;44:1017–1022.

26. Girard DE, Elliot DL, Hickam DH, et al. The internship: A prospective investigation of emotions and attitudes. *West J Med.* 1986;144:93–98.

27. Hendrie HC, Clair DK, Brittain HM, Fadul PE. A study of anxiety/depressive symptoms of medical students, house staff, and their spouses/partners. *J Nerv Ment Dis.* 1990;178:204–207.

28. Ziegler JL, Strull WM, Larsen RC. Stress in medical training—Medical staff conference. University of California, San Francisco. *West J Med.* 1985;142:814–819.

29. Baldwin PJ, Newton RW, Buckley G, Roberts MA, Dodd M. Senior house officers in medicine: Postal survey of training and work experience. *BMJ.* 1997;314:740–743.

30. Samkoff JS, Jacques CHM. A review of studies concerning effects of sleep deprivation and fatigue on residents' performance. *Acad Med.* 1991;66:687–693.

31. Lingenfelser T, Kaschel R, Weber A, Zaiser-Kaschel H, Jakober B, Kuper J. Young hospital doctors after night duty: Their task specific cognitive status and emotional condition. *Med Educ.* 1994;28:566–572.

32. Spurgeon A, Harrington JM. Work performance and health of junior hospital doctors. *Work and Stress.* 1989;3:117–128.

33. Harrington JM. Working long hours and health. *BMJ.* 1994; 308:1581–1582.

34. Goldberg DP, Hillier VF. A scaled version of the General Health Questionnaire. *Psycholog Med.* 1979;9:139–145.

35. Geurts S, Rutte C, Peeters M. Antecedents and consequences of work-home interference among medical residents. *Soc Sci Med.* 1999;48:1135–1148.

36. Baldwin PJ, Dodd M, Wrate RM. Junior doctors making mistakes. *The Lancet.* 1998; 351:804.

37. Firth-Cozens J. Sources of stress and ways of coping in junior house officers. *Stress Med.* 1989;5:121–126.

38. May HJ, Revicki DA. Professional stress among family physicians. *J Fam Pract.* 1985;20:165–170.

39. Silver HK, Glicken AD. Medical student abuse: Incidence, severity, and significance. *JAMA.* 1990;263:527–532.

40. Coombs RH, Fawzy FI. The effect of marital status on stress in medical school. *Am J Psychiatry.* 1982;139:1490–1493.

41. Ford CV, Wentz DK. The internship year: A study of sleep, mood states, and psychophysiologic parameters. *South Med J.* 1984; 77:1435–1442.

42. Landau C, Hall S, Wartman SA, Macko MB. Stress in social and family relationships during the medical residency. *J Med Educ.* 1986;61:654–660.

43. Kelner M, Rosenthal C. Postgraduate medical training, stress, and marriage. *Can J Psychiatry.* 1986;31:22–24.

44. Whitley TW, Gallery ME, Allison EJ Jr, et al. Factors associated with stress among emergency medicine residents. *Ann Emerg Med.* 1989;18:1157–1161.

45. Sotile WM, Sotile MO. Today's medical marriage: Part 1. *JAMA.* 1997;277:1180c.

46. Townsend MH, Wallick MM, Cambre KM. Follow-up survey of support services for lesbian, gay, and bisexual medical students. *Acad Med.* 1996;71:1012–1014.

47. Brogan DJ, Frank E, Elon L, Sivanesan P, O'Hanlan KA. Harassment of lesbians as medical students and physicians. *JAMA*. 1999;282:1290–1292.

48. Ramos MM, Tellez CM, Palley TB, Umland BE, Skipper BJ. Attitudes of physicians practicing in New Mexico toward gay men and lesbians in the profession. *Acad Med*. 1998;73:436–438.

49. Burke BP, White JC. Wellbeing of gay, lesbian, and bisexual doctors. *BMJ*. 2001;322:422.

50. Sotile WM, Sotile MO. *Beat Stress Together: The BEST Way to a Passionate Marriage, A Healthy Family, and a Productive Life*. New York, NY: John Wiley & Sons; 1999.

51. Sotile WM, Sotile MO. *The Medical Marriage: Sustaining Positive Relationships for Physicians and Their Families*, Revised Edition. Chicago, Ill: American Medical Association Press; 2000.

52. Sotile WM, Sotile MO. Today's medical marriage: Part 1. *JAMA*. 1997;277(16):1322.

53. Robinson DO. The medical-student spouse syndrome: Grief reactions to the clinical years. *Am J Psychiatry*. 1978;135:972–974.

54. Pittman F. *Private Lies: Infidelity and Betrayal of Intimacy*. New York, NY: W.W. Norton; 1990.

55. Brown E. *Affairs: A Guide for Working Through the Repercussions of Infidelity*. New York, NY: Jossey-Bass; 1999.

56. Burkhart J. Resident forum: AMA-RPS instrumental in achieving new maternity leave policy. *JAMA*. 1991;265:1756.

57. Sinal S, Weavil P, Camp MG. Survey of women physicians on issues relating to pregnancy during a medical career. *Med Educ*. 1988; 63:531–538.

58. Ducker D. Research on women physicians with multiple roles: A feminist perspective. *JAMWA*. 1994;49:78–84.

59. Bickel J. Maternity leave policies for residents: An overview of issues and problems. *Acad Med*. 1989;64:498–501.

60. Sayres M, Wyshak G, Denterlein G, Apfel R, Shore E, Federman D. Pregnancy during residency. *N Engl J Med*. 1986;314:418–423.

61. Young-Shumate L, Kramer T. Pregnancy during graduate medical training. *Acad Med*. 1993; 68:792.

62. Sells JM, Sells CJ. Pediatrician and patient: A challenge for female physicians. *Pediatr*. 1989;84:355–361.

63. Council of Teaching Hospitals. *Cost Survey of Housestaff Stipends, Benefits and Funding.* Washington, DC: Association of American Medical Colleges; 1989.

64. Klebanoff MA, Shiono PH, Rhoads GG. Spontaneous and induced abortion among resident physicians. *JAMA.* 1991;265:2821.

65. Eskenazi L, Weston J. The pregnant plastic surgical resident: Results of a survey of women plastic surgeons and plastic surgery residency directors. *Plast Reconstr Surg.* 1995;95:330–335.

66. Rogers C, Kunkel ES, Field H. Impact of pregnancy during training on a psychiatric resident cohort. *JAMWA.* 1994;49:49–52.

67. Braun DL, Susman VL. Pregnancy during psychiatry residency: A study of attitudes. *Acad Psychiatry.* 1992;16:178–185.

68. Riley CA, Jagiella V, Michaletz-Onody P, et al. Parental leave for trainees in gastroenterology. *Am J Gastroenterol.* 1992;87:1368–1371.

69. Bernstein AE. Maternity leave for residents. *JAMWA.* 1987;42:70.

70. Little AM. Why can't a woman be more like a man? *N Engl J Med.* 1990;323:1064–1065.

71. Bongiovi ME, Freedman J. Maternity leave experiences of resident physicians. *JAMWA.* 1993;48:185–193.

72. Klebanoff MA, Shiono PH, Rhoads GG. Outcomes of pregnancy in a national sample of resident physicians. *N Engl J Med.* 1990;323:1040–1045.

73. Silva BM. Pregnancy during residency: A look at the issues. *JAMWA.* 1992;47:71–74.

74. Spirit BA, Rauth VA, Price AP, Hayman LA. Pregnancy and maternity leave: AAWR survey results. *Radiol.* 1990;176:325–328.

75. AMA Ad Hoc Committee on Women Physicians. *Maternity Leave for Residents.* Chicago, Ill: American Medical Association; 1984:1–21.

76. Katz VL, Miller NH, et al. Pregnancy complications of physicians. *West J Med.* 1988;149:704.

77. Meijman TF, ed. Workload and recovery: A theoretical framework in work psychological research on workload. In: *Mentale Belasting en Werkstress: een Arbeidspsychologicische Benadering.* Van Gorcum, Assen, pp. 5–20 (Reported in Geurts et al, 1999).

78. Gottlieb DJ, Parenti C, Peterson CA, Lofgren RP. Effect of a change in house staff work schedule on resource utilization and patient care. *Arch Int Med.* 1991;151:2065–2070.

79. Brashear DB. Support groups and other supporting efforts in residency programs. *J Med Educ.* 1987;62:418–424.
80. McCranie EW, Brandsma JM. Personality antecedents of burnout among middle-aged physicians. *Behav Med.* 1988;(Spring):30–36.
81. Mazie B. Job stress, psychological health, and social support of family practice residents. *J Med Educ.* 1985;60:935–941.
82. Frone MR, Russell M, Cooper ML. Antecedents and outcomes of work-family conflict: Testing a model of the work-family interface. *J Appl Psychol.* 1992;77:65–78.
83. Purdy RR, Lemkau JP, Rafferty JP, Rudisill JR. Resident physicians in family practice: Who's burned out and who knows? *Fam Med.* 1987;19:203–208.
84. Lum G, Goldberg R, Mallon WK, Lew B, Margulies J. A survey of wellness issues in emergency medicine (Part 2). *Ann Emerg Med.* 1995;25:242–248.
85. Bell B. Evolutionary imperatives, quiet revolutions: Changing working conditions and supervision of house officers. *The Pharos.* 1989; Spring:16–19.
86. Department of Health. *Hours of Work of Doctors in Training: The New Deal.* London: Department of Health; 1991.
87. Paice E, West G, Cooper R, Orton V, Scotland A. Senior house officer training: Is it getting better? *BMJ.* 1997;314:719–720.
88. Heyworth J, Whitley TW, Allison EJ, Revicki DA. Predictors of work satisfaction among SHOs during accident and emergency medicine training. *Arch Emerg Med.* 1993;10:279–288.
89. Residency Services Committee, Association of Program Directors in Internal Medicine. Stress and impairment during residency training: Strategies for reductions, identification, and management. *Ann Intern Med.* 1988;109:154–161.
90. Moss F, Miller C. Getting the organizational environment right. In: Paice E, ed. *Delivering the New Doctor.* Edinburgh; ASME, 1998;27–32.
91. McCue J. The distress of internship. *N Engl J Med.* 1985;312:449–452.
92. Linn LS, Brook RH, Clark VA, Ross DA. Physician and patient satisfaction as factors related to the organization of internal medicine group practices. *Med Care.* 1985;23:1171—1178.
93. Walker JL, Janssen H, Hubbard D. Gender differences in attrition from orthopaedic surgery residency. *JAMWA.* 1993;48:182–184.

94. Firth-Cozens J. Emotional distress in junior house officers. *BMJ*. 1987;295:533–536.

95. Richardson C. Shadowing: The Leicester experience. In: Paice E, ed. *Delivering the New Doctor*. Edinburgh: ASME; 1998.

96. Levinson DJ, Darrow CN, Klein EM, Levinson MH, McKee B. *Seasons of a Man's Life*. New York, NY: Random House; 1978.

97. Ridson C, Cook D, Willms D. Gay and lesbian physicians in training: A qualitative study. *Can Med Assoc J*. 2000;162:331–334.

98. Randall CJ. Learning medicine through the closet door. *Ann Intern Med*. 1999;131:470.

99. Thompson I. Being a gay medical student. *Student BMJ*. 1998;6:431.

100. Townsend MH, Wallick MM. Gay, lesbian, and bisexual issues in medical schools: Implications for training. In: Cajaj RP, Stein TS, eds. *Textbook of Homosexuality and Mental Health*. Washington, DC: American Psychiatric Press, Inc; 1996.

101. Schneider JS, Levin S. Uneasy partners: The lesbian and gay health care community and the AMA. *JAMA*. 1999;282:1287.

102. Giordano J, McGoldrick M, Pearce JK, eds. *Ethnicity & Family Therapy*. New York, NY: Guilford Press; 1996.

103. Oyama ON. Investigating the influence of peer-group cohesion on residents' levels of stress and performance at two residencies. *Acad Med*. 1991; June, 66:371.

104. Mushin IC, Matteson MT, Lynch EC. Developing a resident assistance program: Beyond the support group model. *Arch Intern Med*. 1993;153:729–733.

105. Matthews DA, Classen DC, Willms JL, Cotton JP. A program to help interns cope with stresses in an internal medicine residency. *J Med Educ*. 1988;63:539–547.

106. Kahn NB, Addison RB. Comparison of support services offered by residencies in six specialties, 1979–80, and 1988–89. *Acad Med*. 1992;67:197–202.

107. Samuel SS, Lawrence JS, Schwartz HJ, Weiss JC, Seltzer JL. Investigating stress levels of residents: A pilot study. *Med Teacher*. 1991;13:89–92.

108. Shapiro SL, Schwartz GE, Bonner G. Effects of mindfulness-based stress reduction on medical and premedical students. *J Behav Med*. 1998;21:581–599.

109. Kling PJ, Fost N. A faculty-house staff retreat. *Amer J of Dis Child.* 1992;146:242–248.

110. Mygdal WK, Monteiro M, Hitchcock M, Featherston W, Conrad S. Outcomes of the first family practice chief resident leadership conference. *Fam Med.* 1991;23:308–310.

111. McCue JD, Sachs CL. A stress management workshop improves residents' coping skills. *Arch Intern Med.* 1991;151:2273–2277.

112. Kaplan C, Marshall M. Sources of resistance to an intern support group. *J Med Educ.* 1988;63:906–911.

chapter 13

Making Your Workplace a Positive Interpersonal Culture

"There is virtually no relationship between being an expert and being seen as someone people can trust with their secrets, doubts, and vulnerabilities."

Daniel Goleman
Emotional Intelligence[1]

Do the following symptoms of an unhealthy medical workplace[2] describe your office, hospital, or organization?

- Persistent blaming and complaining
- Low morale and high burnout
- High turnover
- Poorly expressed frustration and anger
- Difficulty in recruiting
- Minimal demonstration of appreciation
- People not liking to come to work
- Absenteeism
- Inefficient, ineffective, and/or nonexistent meetings
- Frequent policy changes
- Overt or covert threats
- Difficulty in planning vacations or time off

If so, you and the people around you are probably suffering professionally, emotionally, and physically. Let us elaborate.

The wealth of empirical and clinical research presented in this book suggests robust cross-correlations between the six factors summarized in Table 13-1. We propose that the interplay between these factors largely determines resilience for physicians and medical organizations.

T A B L E   13-1

The Crucial Interplay

Job and Career Satisfaction Levels of Physicians and Medical Staff

Self-Rated Levels of Personal Happiness

Quality of Marriage and Family Life for Physicians

Physician Health

Patient Ratings of the Quality of Their Medical Care

Patient Ratings of Their Levels of Satisfaction with Their Medical Care

Patient Adherence to Medical Interventions

Rates of Malpractice Claims

Staff Morale

Rates of Retention of Key Employees in the Medical Workplace

We specifically call attention here to the fact that dissatisfaction with work has been shown to correlate with both psychosocial and medical problems, while job satisfaction seems to have fortifying properties. It appears that a supportive work environment not only makes for happier employees and more satisfied patients, it also has health-enhancing benefits.

Clearly, team-building is one of most useful organizational interventions to improve morale and productivity in the workplace and to ensure the mental and physical health of employees.[3] Heyworth and colleagues[4] reported that residents in emergency medicine who view their work groups as cohesive appeared more satisfied with their jobs and less stressed than those who experienced less group cohesiveness. Other researchers, including Carter and West,[5] demonstrated how members of work groups characterized by positive teamwork evidenced enhanced coping, more job satisfaction, less strain, and improved scores on measures of mental health. One specific product is a more cheerful nursing staff, one of the factors that correlates with patient satisfaction.[6]

Finally, research at the University of California at Irvine suggested that informal social support systems at work may be especially important to men's health.[7] This may be due to the fact that many men seem to find it difficult to maintain friendships outside of work, something women approach with more diligence and success. Males, on the other hand, tend to be more dependent on workplace relationships for their social contact.

F I G U R E   13-1

The Stress-Resilient System

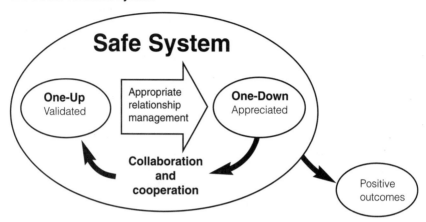

Source: Sotile WM, Sotile MO. Conflict Management: Part 1. How to shape positive
relationships in medical practices and hospitals. *The Physician Executive* 1999;25(4):57-61.
Used with permission.

If ever there were a time to shape medical organizations into
positive interpersonal cultures, now is that time. As depicted in
Figure 13-1, collegiality and collaboration serve as the corner-
stones of a stress-resilient medical organization.[8]

We previously mentioned the unfortunate fact that fewer than
half of physicians polled feel adequately trained in skills needed
to promote collegiality and collaboration—EEM skills like communication and conflict management. It is no wonder that a
study of stress and job satisfaction among 1,817 physicians from
the United Kingdom[9] concluded with the recommendation that

> "consideration should be given to providing general practitioners with more
> time management, people management, and work organisation skill develop-
> ment, as this might well help them to overcome some of the daily and chronic
> stressors of their job."[9 (p. 370)]

The purpose of this chapter is to demonstrate how medical organizations can be transformed into positive, resilient cultures and to
specify the team-building behaviors needed by physician leaders
in the twenty-first century. We start with our conceptual scheme
for how medical organizations develop and grow. This conceptualization is based on observations made during our work with
medical group practices. However, it can be modified to fit most

organizations. Viewing your organization from a developmental perspective can show you the most adaptive and effective *next* steps in you organization's unfolding life cycle. Before elaborating this framework, we offer a caveat.

We emphasize that here, as with all conceptual schemata, the map is not the territory. No theory can fully and accurately represent the experiences of any living, developing human system. At their best, such models provide road maps that give individuals and organizations hope—the belief that they have or will develop the resources they need to accomplish their goals. The purpose of our model is to stimulate your thinking and insights. For newly formed medical groups, this framework can help by highlighting potholes in the road ahead that you can miss only through collaboration. For others, these concepts may stir a retrospective analysis that helps explain how you got into the difficulties you encountered or may still be suffering.

HOW DID WE GET HERE?

As the twentieth century drew to a close, a new age in medicine was in full bloom. Among the many changes was the growth of rapidly forming, hybrid medical organizations. Groups of relatively independent players began to join forces to create large group practices or smaller practices began joining already existing, large medical organizations.

As the days of solo or "mom-and-pop" medical practices draw to a close, physicians who may have grown accustomed to functioning as individuals—those same physicians who say, overwhelmingly, that they were not trained to be effective collaborators, communicators, or managers—now face the mandate to learn how to work together in complex corporations. Many are fraught with ambivalence as they join or form complex medical organizations. Lack of organizational training combined with ambivalence about merging or working for a large corporation sets the stage for problems to develop.[10]

If mismanaged, the interpersonal dynamics in a new organization will strangle morale and productivity. Moving beyond conflict starts with understanding how these problems developed.

Stage I: The New Organization Is Created

Many medical practices morph quickly into existence without the benefit of a corporate "holding ground" or structure to buffer their growing pains. If the new corporate entity lacks appropriate infrastructure and leadership to assure smooth operations,[10] an unstable merger is borne.

Across industries in the United States, the success rate of mergers is only 30% to 60%.[11] The Bureau of Business Research study of 45 Forbes 500 companies reported that organizational and cultural problems are more likely than financial factors to sink a merger. Specifically, mergers have been found to fail for the following reasons:[11,12]

- Key talent leaves
- Lowered overall productivity and individual performance
- Poor communications
- Placement errors
- Key workforce problems are denied, ignored, or mismanaged
- Lack of direction during implementation of the "window of opportunity"
- Ignoring the "culture fit"
- Poor management of remaining employees

Looking over this list, it is clear that mismanaged people issues often make the difference in determining a merger's success or failure. Typically, the people issues are addressed inadequately and at the last minute. The resultant "clash of assumptions, values, and behaviors brought by the people" fosters resentment, lack of cooperation, or chaos.[11]

In the early stage of a medical organization's development, four mistakes are especially likely to occur. We refer to them as the 4 U's:

- Uneven dealings with others
- Unresolved differences
- Unclear definitions
- Letting "Undiscussables" accumulate

*U*neven Dealings With Others

Here, attempts to placate certain colleagues or natural affinity for some colleagues and not others leads to the development of real or perceived factions within the organization. In a prior publication,[8] we presented the following case vignette that demonstrated how this might occur:

> Dr Jones, the elected physician executive of a 16-member, multispecialty practice, came under attack by the group's non-Caucasian members. He was accused of failing to evenly share crucial information with all partners and of overaligning himself with the former group leader, whom the non-Caucasian partners considered to be a racist. Perplexed by the accusation, Dr Jones explained, "I had no idea that this was happening. I do meet frequently with our former group president, but this is simply because I need his input regarding group policies and medical/political issues. Plus, I have assumed that it is my job to lead our practice without bothering every partner with the minutiae of everyday practice business. Now I'm accused of being a racist and of withholding information!"[8 (p. 59)]

Uneven dealings also stem from interpersonal preferences. The comments of Dr X make this point:

> "We are talking about disbanding one of the most successful group practices in the country, all because we can't get along with each other! How in the world did we get here? We're stuck in an 'us versus them' battle that is killing this organization. I swear, I believe that this all started innocently enough. As I see it, here's the deal: Some of us have known each other for years. It's only natural, therefore, that we would continue those friendships, even though we are now a part of a larger group. There has been no conspiracy to harm group morale; we were just continuing our friendships.
>
> "It sure was a lot simpler when we were in our original, small practices. Building relationships with your partners just seemed to happen naturally then, the result of working side-by-side in the trenches every day, trying to stay afloat. Now, we have to worry about the implications of going out to dinner with friends!"

Real or perceived factions can weaken a newly formed medical organization. At a time when group morale needs to solidify from fair, even dealings between all parties, the group's foundation is weakened by crevices that interfere with teamwork.

When practices merge, threats to teamwork come in many guises, including the following:[11]

- Conflicts in corporate cultures
- Unclear reporting structure

- Clashing egos or management styles
- Inadequate or untimely communications
- Poor benefits planning and follow-through
- Unfocused team building
- Inadequate realignment efforts
- Slow pace of integration
- Retention problems

Getting it right from the start. From the outset of a new organization, plan for success by thinking about the "fit" of the players and what needs to happen to boost their morale and retain them as productive group members. All employees must be engaged in and aligned with the new organization's vision. Right Management Consultants recommend that the following points be kept in mind in order to manage the "people factor:"[11]

- *In most medical practice mergers, at least one party feels that it has been "acquired" by a larger, more aggressive or successful group.* Remember that there is a marked difference between the experience and perceptions of those who are acquired and those who are acquiring. The members of the acquiring organizations are 12% more likely to report their experience as a success than those who were acquired.[11] On the other hand, the acquired are likely to feel disenfranchised. Stay mindful of the fact that, before the merger, all parties were "stars" in their own right, at least in some ways. Their ways of doing things (eg, their ways of handling billing, work flow, managing staff, etc) must be honored, even though they may not be adopted. Don't make promises you can't keep. You will not necessarily choose to adopt the other group's ways of doing business. But either lack of respect or lack of clarity about this issue can lead to a sense of resentment and betrayal.
- *Pick your partners carefully.* Evaluate the "cultures" that you are joining. Just like a marriage, a merged medical practice must have shared values and goals if it is to succeed. Here, it pays to be a good listener and a good integrator of the other party's needs. Be sensitive to the other side's feelings.
- *Develop an integration team that plays devil's advocate.* Anticipate as many integration issues as you can brainstorm and develop contingency plans for dealing with each. This involves more

than information systems, billing, and other "hard" aspects of business. Again, remember the people issues. How will egos mesh or clash? Who expects the new organization to function like "one big, interactive, happy family" and who expects to function as a lone wolf left alone to do patient care and little else? In a large group, there may be room enough for all styles. But be realistic here.

- *Be realistic about how you are going to run the new organization.* Develop a detailed plan of how you are going to merge the organizations, how you are going to deal with cultural differences, and how you are going to communicate with employees.

- *Remember that most people are frightened by change.* Your integration plan needs to accept this as a fact that will play a major role in influencing group dynamics, especially during the initial stages of organizational life. Employees and colleagues will have to be helped to adopt a shared vision of how the new organization will benefit them. Remember that "nobody concentrates on anything until their 'me' issues are resolved."[11 (p. 17)] Personal concerns will prompt people to align with leaders who make them feel safe, even if doing so works against the creation of team unity in the new organization.

- *Never underestimate the importance of sharing information.* The more the people in your organization understand what the new practice looks and feels like for them, the more comfortable and productive they will become. Provide employees with formal or informal career coaching that helps them see the merger as an opportunity. In the event that the merger will result in job loss, provide outplacement counseling.

- *Proactively build up the survivors.* Don't assume that surviving the merger is benefit enough for your employees. Remember: People quit jobs based on feeling undervalued, dead-ended, and unnurtured, not just for financial reasons. Find out what motivates your staff and colleagues (eg, attention, encouragement, involvement in decision making, acknowledgment, appreciation) and give it to them.

- *Be humble.* Mergers create larger organizations that are more resilient than individuals can be. No one is irreplaceable. Set standards and insist that everyone adhere to them (eg, codes of conduct, noncompete agreements, rotations for remote clinics). Remember that the leaders' behaviors set the tone for a merger.

- *Take advantage of the window of opportunity to shape positive teamwork.* Systems in flux reorganize rather quickly. Attend diligently to team- and morale-building practices during the first year of operations. Emphasize from the outset that participation in team-building meetings and activities is an expected part of belonging to this new group. Solo players need not apply.

- *Accept that this is a process, not an event.* Building a new organization takes time. You must accumulate shared experiences, communicate and problem solve effectively, and honor each other if you are to create a dynamic, resilient organization.

Unresolved Differences

Team building takes effort, skill, and *regularly setting aside time to meet and discuss your affairs.* Various factors converge to put busy medical groups at risk of omitting this last, crucial ingredient in the formula for team building.

First, most medical groups are so bombarded with demands on physician time that staging regular business meetings may seem like an unacceptable intrusion in already stressed work–family juggling acts. Second, medical groups seldom have a human resource professional who is both empowered and credentialed to keep track of the group's interpersonal dynamics. Finally, as we stated earlier, when it comes to their conflict-management style, physicians, like many high-powered copers, tend to follow the "hit-and-run" model.[13,14]

All of these factors may combine to result in a tacit group decision to "skip" attending to this prerequisite for team building—regular attendance and participation in group meetings. If meetings do not occur, the group will inevitably accumulate tensions related to unresolved conflict. Beware of this trap. Problem dynamics that would fizzle if addressed directly will fester if neglected.

The accumulated tensions that come with unresolved conflicts set the stage for the emergence of a second syndrome that signals struggling organizational development. Here, a delegated or self-appointed "peacemaker" emerges. This person attempts to soothe brewing conflict by assuming the role of shuttle diplomat: He or she speaks to party A about problems or concerns regarding party B, does the same with party B about party A, but fails to facilitate parties A and B dealing directly and productively with each other. In so doing, the peacemaker actually becomes part of the problem.

Such buffering interactions, no mater how well-intended, can interfere with what is most needed at this stage of the organization's development: Direct dealings between partners that will foster the trust and teamwork needed in order to grow and mature.

Unclear Definitions

During times of change, medical organizations may fail to specify behavioral expectations that will guide the organizational culture. In the absence of such guidelines, important questions fill the minds of the organization's membership.[15] Failing to answer these questions stirs resistance to change. Openly addressing the following factors diminishes resistance to change and fuels cooperation, collaboration, and team-building:

- Why should I believe that this change is really needed?
- Will I be involved in the planning related to the change?
- Will I receive ample communication about the change?
- How will this communicating take place?
- What are the facts that led to this change being made?
- How will I be affected by this change?
- How might I be recognized and/or rewarded related to this change?
- What new behavior will be expected of me in the wake of this change?
- What are the potential benefits of this change for the organization, for our medical community, for my patients, and for myself?
- Will support be available during crunch time when we are learning and/or perfecting new and/or different skills related to this change? If so, in what form(s) will this support be offered?
- Is any particular information or training needed for making this change successfully, both in advance and during the change process?
- Can I trust the individual or team leading the change?
- Are the people in charge of spearheading this change serious about this being a necessary and adaptive change?
- From logistical and physical standpoints, how will this change affect my work life?
- Is there an interesting challenge in this change?

- What would happen if we did not implement this change?
- What are the best-case consequences and/or the possibilities that may come with this change?
- Where are the matches between this change and my own personal career goals?
- How might this change provide me with more interesting (or career-enhancing) work?
- What breakdowns are likely to happen during the crunch time of implementing the change?
- How will we go about problem solving when breakdowns happen?

This list of questions can serve several purposes. First, it can be used to stimulate group discussion and problem-solving related to any organizational change. It can also guide you as you assess your personal reactions to an anticipated change. Finally, these questions can structure your one-on-one dealings with colleagues or employees concerned about a proposed or upcoming change. In each case, the questions can stimulate all parties concerned to discuss their thoughts and feelings and to specify what information they need in order to get on board with the change.

A variant of the "unclear definitions" that plague many medical groups has to do with their failure to adopt a code of conduct. Even the most visionary medical leader may fear that spearheading such an effort will stir unnecessary conflict; therefore, they avoid this important issue altogether. We extensively discussed this issue in Chapter 9. Here we simply emphasize that the absence of appropriate policies and procedures governing behavior leaves a medical organization attempting to function like a ship at sea without the benefit of a guiding rudder.

Letting "Undiscussables" Accumulate

The fourth "U" in our formula comes when tensions that stem from dysfunctional interpersonal dynamics accumulate and foster what Ryan and Oestreich[16] called "undiscussables." These are issues or facts that everyone knows about but tacitly agrees not to openly discuss. Silence allows the issues to fester, making them more potent than they would otherwise be. Soon, the negative emotions that come from the undiscussables lead to loss of energy, enthusiasm, creativity, and teamwork. Here is an example of how this might occur.

Practice ABC consisted of nine physician-partners ranging in age from mid-30s to mid-60s. The older partners privately grumbled to each other about how disgruntled they were that the younger partners refuse to work as hard as they did early in their own careers. The younger partners were well aware of the grumblings about their work ethic, but they were also steadfast in their commitment to maintain a manageable lifestyle. Failure to openly discuss these issues lead to an "us against them" dynamic in the group that was manifested in various ways that were detrimental to all parties. For example, when partners from different generations shared on-call duties, passive–aggressive reactions to each other predominated. And group issues requiring votes by shareholders led to a predictable generational division of votes. The palpable lack of compassion for each generation's career-management concerns, coupled with silence about the "elephants in the living room," created a serious schism in this group's collegiality.

The good news is that the tensions that come with "undiscussables" tend to immediately lessen once the issues are accurately labeled and appropriately discussed, *even if no ready-made solutions become apparent.* Your experiences in personal relationships probably prove this point.

For example, couples often grow tired of having the same argument about a given topic, like differences in sex drive, differences in parenting style, or differences in money management strategies. They may then begin to avoid discussing the topic. The tensions that develop from treating the topic like an "undiscussable" simply serve to magnify each person's privately held thoughts and feelings about the problem. Soon, one or both mates may fear that this issue is relationship threatening. Finally, an open "discussion" (ie, argument) erupts. What happens next tends to be liberating. Even though the differences that led to the syndrome are still in place, both parties now feel a palpable degree of relief. The "undiscussable" was discussed, thereby rendering the issue relatively inert. The power of the problem issue starts to pale in comparison to the powerful ways your relationship grows as you make sincere efforts to problem-solve and communicate, *even if the problem is not solved.*

Stage II: The Disjointed Organization Develops

If variants of the 4 U's just outlined are left unchecked, discontent with the organization and its leadership grows. You know this is happening when the "silent majority" grows restless. Remember that most physicians—even those who may not have asserted

themselves as leaders from the outset of this new organization—
tend to share a common characteristic: They are high-powered,
self-directed, opinionated people. In our experience, the charismatic individual or the "inner circle" of physicians who assume
initial leadership of a group inevitably come under fire from this
silent majority.

What happens next is a subtle shift in the group's interpersonal
dynamic, one that works against the very factors the organization
most needs at this stage of growth—group cohesion and collegiality.
The emergence of "team-killer" behaviors like those listed following[16] signal that your organization has become a disjointed system:

- Factions develop and stop speaking to each other
- Differences lead to disagreements that fester into conflicts
- Intragroup competition for status, referrals, or power flourishes
- Partners begin to gossip about each other
- Incidents of inappropriate or unprofessional behavior escalate
- Passive–aggressive ploys become commonplace, including
  failing to attend important group business meetings, refusing
  to embrace the spirit of policies that would otherwise improve
  practice operations, and/or showing disregard or discourtesy
  to certain colleagues within the group
- Communication between partners fills with silences, brevity,
  and abruptness
- Certain physicians feel snubbed or ignored by others
- Implied or stated insults creep into group discussions
- Through acts of omission or commission, partners discredit or
  discount each other's contributions to the practice
- When things go wrong, blaming becomes the most common
  mode of response
- Secretive decision making and lobbying begins to pervade the
  group process
- Defensiveness rather than acceptance becomes the most typical
  response to feedback
- Direct feedback between physicians ceases and is replaced by
  mixed messages
- Cold, aloof behavior becomes standard

At this point, an interesting ambivalence about changing tends
to paralyze the group.[10] How the group goes about using and

responding to organizational consultants is one manifestation of this ambivalence.

During this stage, consultants are often called in at the cost of considerable time and money. But the group's ambivalence about their desired direction of change results in an interesting paradox: They employ the consultant, but do not follow his or her advice. In our experience, this is due to two factors.

First, not all members of the group are at the same stage of the change paradigm outlined in Chapter 11. Some members, having steadfastly observed the negative decline in the group, are at the Action stage. They are ready to respond to helpful input about new ways of structuring and managing the group dynamics and the group's business.

Other group members may be floundering at the Precontemplation, Contemplation, or Preparation stages. They either have not yet taken seriously the need to change anything about the status quo (Precontemplation) or they are noticing problems but are not yet ready to take action (Contemplation or Preparation). Typically, these are the group members who simply have not paid much attention to the organization's dynamics. They heretofore have been content to simply do their work and get home as soon as they can. They have shown little interest in dealing with any business demands that require their time.

Also underlying the hire-and-ignore-consultants syndrome is ambivalence about giving up power. Let us elaborate.

As a new organization's foundation is weakened by "cracks" in group cohesion caused by schisms and coalitions between partners, a certain type of leader tends to emerge. Here, the person with the most charismatic style, extraverted personality, political savvy, and/or sheer will and willingness to spend time and effort running the company will take control. As long as the group functions in relative disarray, such leaders wield power. If the group grows more cohesive, however, the "cracks" in the organization disappear, and this type of leader loses power. Herein lies fuel for the paradox about employing but not following the advice of consultants.

We have developed an adage suggested by our experiences as consultants to medical organizations at this stage in their journey: The one who hires you will be the first one to want to fire you. Why? Because, if a consultant is doing his or her job, group cohesion and teamwork improve, and the leader whose empowerment is dependent upon the organization's *lack* of cohesion is threatened by the consultant's input.

The Loneliness of Medical Leaders

We are often struck by the pain that medical leaders experience at the hands of their colleagues. This is nowhere more apparent than in maturing medical groups. At first, the newly forming group is appreciative that someone is doing the relatively thankless "in-the-trenches" work of leading the new organization. But this same leader eventually becomes the target of discontents that seem inevitably to grow in a group of independent thinkers who value autonomy.

What results is a no-win situation for the early leader. If others hold back from taking the reins, the charismatic leader may continue to lead by default. But as the silent majority begins to speak up, the very person who assumed or was assigned the role of leader during the group's formation will be targeted as a threat to the organization's growth. Fair or not, developing organizations tend to eventually accuse their early leaders of being manipulative, duplicitous, controlling, and/or egomaniacal. If mismanaged, this process can prove to be extremely costly to both the organization and the individuals involved.

Any physician or organization that is undergoing this dynamic is in pain. It is helpful for medical groups to heed a lesson learned from corporate America. Collins and Porras[17] studied "visionary companies," those known to be premiere within their industries. They noted that, among other things, these resilient companies are driven to change and to improve; and, if they grow appropriately, they become capable of continued success *without being dependent on one great idea or one charismatic leader.*

In our consultation, we emphasize the importance of embracing what has been good and right about the decisions that have driven the organization's journey thus far while also accepting that transition to new styles of leadership will periodically be necessary if the organization is to continue growing. Take care to express appreciation for the contributions of each member of your organization every step along your journey and work to keep perspective. Similar to families, organizations grow; with that growth comes the need for change and flexibility, never blame and resentment.

Stage III: A New Crisis Threatens

Often, a new, high-stakes crisis signals entry into Stage III of our developmental schema. The nature of this crisis tends to reflect both what is wrong with the group and what needs to be done to promote more group cohesion.

Here, the dysfunctional aspects of the group's interpersonal dynamics foster symptoms of intragroup discord. These symptoms might initially take the forms of passive or passive–aggressive acts, such as failure to attend group meetings. But Stage III is signaled by a bona fide crisis that involves blatant, even dramatic, demonstrations of conflict. What follows are actual examples drawn from our consulting experiences of just how bad things can get at this stage of organizational development:

- Provider contracts with hospitals or third-party carriers may be canceled due to the fact that the medical group has failed to control the boorish behavior of certain of their physician partners.
- Factions within the group may threaten to splinter off and create competition for the mother practice.
- Individual physicians may threaten to sue certain of their partners and/or the organization for harassment, slander, discrimination, or failure to correct a hostile work environment.
- Partners may engage in open conflict, dramatic arguments, or even fist fights.
- Within-group conflicts may become public, with partners openly disparaging each other or arguing in front of colleagues and the hospital community.

When such crises threaten to disintegrate the group, consultants often are called back in. This time, the groups respond differently. They begin to openly discuss the "undiscussables," and greater cohesion and teamwork begins to manifest.

This increased group cohesiveness weeds out those physicians who are not interested in being team players. Now, behaviors that have gone unnoticed or tolerated stand in stark contrast to the mode of operating that the group is adopting and insisting upon. An example of what can happen follows:

John was chronically ambivalent about whether he would remain a member of his large, multidiscipline group practice or spearhead the formation of a splinter group. He acted shocked when he was confronted by his colleagues about the fact that he was the only partner who had not yet signed a newly revised group employment agreement that specified a behavioral code prohibiting physicians from making disparaging remarks about each other to valued referral sources. He objected, "I've been working here for the past 4 years without a signed employment agreement. How was I supposed to know that we now are taking this stuff seriously?"

Stage IV: Participatory Reorganizing

Stage IV begins as the group moves to revamp its leadership. Now, as physician partners begin to take seriously the need for full participation in organizational meetings and functions, both the structure and the process of the group may be changed. Signs of passive resistance to the organization's rules, regulations, and mores begin to diminish. Many groups at this stage conclude that it would be a mistake to assume that their complex organization can continue to effectively be run by part-time volunteer help of already overworked partners. In today's environment, it is virtually impossible for an already-busy physician to effectively administrate and lead the organization while also maintaining full clinical caseloads.

Groups have several options here. They might choose to hire and/or empower a full-fledged group CEO, manager, or physician executive. At the same time, many move toward management by committee. At minimum, the independence and influence of individual leaders is tempered by the formation or activation of a group executive committee that becomes more involved in actual decision making.

The choice of new leadership is most often based on what the group needs in order to foster more positive and powerful collegiality. For example, if issues of trust and fairness have eroded group cohesion, the group will tend to empower those colleagues who are perceived to be the least egocentric and most even-handed in their dealings with others, even if those individuals are not among the most senior or politically savvy partners in the group.

If group credibility has been compromised by inappropriate, disruptive physician behaviors, new leaders who are experienced, respected, and powerful enough to spearhead confrontation of misbehaving partners will be chosen. Or, if the main threat to the group is economic viability, those partners who have the most business savvy may gain leadership status.

At this juncture, many groups shift from a hierarchical leadership structure (in which only a few physicians hold information
and the corresponding power it brings) to a more complimentary
leadership structure—one that allows a more diffuse distribution
of information and decision-making power. The group may
expand from one to two governing committees that function with
equal degrees of autonomy and power. One serves as the group's
executive committee and is charged with the responsibility of
making business-related decisions. The second committee is
charged with managing human resource issues. Both committees
report directly to the organization's board of directors, which typically consists of all physicians who are full partners in the practice.

This second committee is conceptualized variously by different
groups. A few examples we have encountered follow: risk management committee, internal affairs committee, group improvement
committee, group cohesion committee, behavioral affairs committee, human resources committee, and collegiality committee.

Regardless of its name, this second committee is charged
with monitoring and intervening to correct any behavioral or
interpersonal problems that may violate the group's code of
conduct or otherwise threaten morale, teamwork, or operations.
Often, attempts are made to have the organization's executive
committee or its board of directors perform these functions. We
do not recommend this. Consultants generally agree that if a
group's executive committee or its board of directors tries to add
the role of monitoring professional behavior to its already
burgeoning list of responsibilities, the behavioral issues will be
ignored in deference to ever-urgent business items.

The composition of this monitoring committee will depend on
the level of trust and the amount of conflict present in the group.[18]
If the group has a high level of trust and a low level of conflict, a
committee that consists exclusively of physician partners may
work. But if trust is low and conflict is high, the committee
should incorporate trusted individuals from outside the practice.
One example is a committee consisting of the practice manager, a
selected physician, an attorney, and a human resource consultant.
As one physician of a struggling group practice explained to us:

"If we trusted each other to be fair, we probably wouldn't have needed your consultation in the first place. The problem is, we *don't* trust each other. I know that I
wouldn't trust any of my partners enough to give them the power to evaluate and

deal with behavioral issues. And I doubt that any of them trust me that much, either. Too much has happened in this group. We need the input of people who can stay objective; people who don't have personal agendas or scores to settle with any of us."

Whatever its makeup, it is crucial that this committee be empowered to function independently and in parallel to other governing bodies that report directly to the organization's board of directors. The committee should specifically be empowered to investigate, counsel, and discipline violators.

The Maturing Medical Organization

With these two committees in place—one managing business, one managing behaviors—groups typically begin to solidify and mature at a rapid rate. Decisions are more easily made and implemented; "undiscussables" are not allowed to accumulate and fester; and, if nothing else, through the sheer act of regularly meeting and encountering each other, greater levels of collegiality and collaboration begin to develop. The signs of these positive changes are outlined here[19]:

Collegiality is signaled by:

- Acknowledgment of interdependence
- "You do what you want, and I'll do what I want" attitude of acceptance
- Heightened sense of autonomy and independence
- Respect shown for individual differences in training and practice methods
- "You don't monitor or criticize me, and I won't monitor or criticize you" attitude

Collaboration is signaled by:

- Free exchange of information and help within the group
- Acknowledgment of a common vision, mission, and business purpose
- Open requests for help from colleagues within the organization
- Speaking with a single voice, especially to parties outside the organization
- Holding each other accountable for behaviors that affect integration and interdependence

As can be seen from the above descriptions, the behaviors that signal collegiality and collaboration can sometimes seem contradictory. For example, at once calling for respect of individual differences and communally monitored standards of behavior. This paradox in a small way mirrors the more general difficulty physicians face in today's changing world of medicine.

CHARACTERISTICS OF TEAM-BUILDING MEDICAL LEADERS

To many physicians, the notion of devoting time and energy to "team building" is foreign, if not downright offensive. When we are asked to consult with medical groups having interpersonal difficulties, one faction inevitably takes the position, "Why can't everyone just show up with their 'game face' on and do the job? Life in medicine is complicated enough these days. Now you're telling me that I've got to become some sort of 'human relations' expert? Give me a break!"

As difficult a pill as it may be to swallow, the truth is that the twenty-first century's successful physician *does* need to develop and use effective human relations skills. Unfortunately, physicians—especially senior physicians—tend to greatly underestimate both the positive and negative effects they can have on others in the workplace.[20] Remember these crucial facts, which were mentioned earlier.

- Approximately 65% of nurses claim that they are verbally abused by physicians at least once every 2 to 3 months[21]
- Forty-six percent of those who quit their jobs do so because they feel unappreciated[16]
- Among white-collar workers, inept criticism is the most prevalent cause of conflict on the job[22]

A checklist of approaches taken by team-building medical leaders follows. This list integrates our own observations with those of many authors who have written about leadership in business organizations:[1,11,16,23,24]

- Recognize that the leadership style that got you here may not work in the new organization.
- Become a master of coping with change.

- During times of organizational change, be sure to attend to the following tasks:

  Get full commitment to the plan

  Communicate a unified purpose

  Coach key players to manage transition and conflict

  Openly discuss the positive case for any proposed change, both on a personal and professional level

  Promote understanding of the change process

- Hold regular, focused meetings that include all principals in your organization.

- Communicate, communicate, communicate.

- Openly and evenly share information with your partners.

- Work to include your entire group in decision-making processes.

- Do not participate in gossip or coalitions within your group. Respect colleagues' rights to confidentiality without contributing to triangular patterns of communication. Instead, encourage partners who may be having difficulty with each other to meet and discuss their concerns.

- Facilitate regular meetings to discuss "undiscussables," using the following ground rules:

  Everyone speaks for himself/herself

  Don't interrupt the speaker

  Be specific regarding concerns

  Remember that the purpose of this discussion is to identify work-related problems in order to move forward together, not to place blame

  Let statements lead to requests for change

  If confused, paraphrase and ask for clarification

- Effectively coordinate teamwork.

- Openly praise and express appreciation to each of your physician partners.

- Show that you are proud to be a member of this organization. Speak positively about the work of the people in your group and of your organization as a whole.

- Verbalize optimism about the future.

- Work to build consensus.

- Give others credit for their good work.
- Frequently express gratitude to others in your workplace.
- Speak in terms of "we" rather than creating "us-and-them" distinctions.
- Verbalize insights from the perspective of other physicians, nurses, and administrators.
- Model how to offer constructive criticism.
- Role model taking responsibility, rather than making excuses or blaming others.
- Model the give-and-take of constructive criticism.
- Show initiative to take on responsibilities above and beyond your stated job.
- Don't waste energy trying to find ways to cut corners. Try to find ways to accomplish more.
- Focus on what you do well and, where possible, delegate what you are not good at doing.
- Demonstrate self-management by regulating your time and work commitments and avoid the assumption of a martyred position.
- Collaborate on important issues.
- Focus on common purposes and do not get sidetracked by differences in the details.
- Respect organizational structures and roles and do not use them in undermining ways.
- Never act like you are the exception to the rules that govern the group.
- Admit your own shortcomings and mistakes.
- In front of others, solicit the opinions and input of other physician-partners. Ask for help and express appreciation when you get it. Regularly admit, "I'm not good at doing this, could you help me out?" Then frequently express appreciation to those whose talents are different from your own. Remember: What they do makes it possible for you not to have to do it.
- Stay curious. Expanding your skills and knowledge is one way to rejuvenate your interest and passion for your work.
- Let others know when you are enjoying yourself. Learn to enjoy doing the work involved in your job. Show passion for what you do.

- Take responsibility for the effects that your actions have on others.
- Celebrate! Catch yourself and others doing stuff right; acknowledge positive changes and collaborative efforts shown by others.
- Apologize frequently.
- Give others the benefit of the doubt. Doing so builds trust.
- Regularly inquire about and show regard for the family of each of your colleagues.
- Express appreciation of each other's background and experience.

Within-group interactions need to demonstrate respect for the fact that one's colleagues are more than physicians; they are people who have diverse lives. And today's medical groups are culturally diverse with reference to gender, age, and ethnicity. For example, more than 40% of physicians in internal medicine residency training programs are foreign born.[25] It is human nature to feel most affinity for people who respect and understand the complexity of your life, who see your work role within the larger context of your totality.

At minimum, it is important to express an interest in learning about each other's families, heritage, and traditions. This will only happen if, individually and as a group, you make it a priority to initiate conversations and experiences that allow you to expand your perspectives on each other.

Remember that practices mature as a function of two factors: the passage of time and the accumulated by-products of interactions between group members.

We have found it to be of particular value for medical colleagues to periodically interact with each other in settings other than work. Herein lies the team-building value of staging yearly practice retreats, office holiday celebrations, or casual social affairs that bring your families together. Seeing a colleague in new contexts expands your perceptions of that individual; you now see him or her not only as a physician-colleague but as a person—someone who has a spouse, children, interests, and abilities outside of medicine, even a sense of humor. Such experiences serve to build traditions that will deepen your collegial relationships and mature your organization. Doing so also makes it more likely that when you have conflict with each other in the workplace, you will respond to each other as individuals worthy of mutual positive regard, rather than as adversaries.

EEM TRAINING FOR MEDICAL GROUPS

One of the most helpful and realistic attitudes to foster in any medical organization is that change, disagreement, and periods of conflict are inevitable. Stress-hardy organizations inoculate themselves from the potential toxic effects of these factors. To do so, Marcus et al[26] recommended that you consider the following series of questions:

- What are the potential disputes that we may encounter down the road?
- How are we going to resolve those issues so they cause minimal disruption for operations and minimal drain on the budget?
- What can we do to manage the conflicts that do occur?
- How can we change or rearrange the organization to reduce the likelihood of conflict?
- What will we do to learn from these disputes and then appropriately adjust our procedures to lessen the likelihood that the problem will recur?

We encourage you to commit to making your medical workplace a healthy one. Regardless of your work setting, this mission can be aided by offering workplace training and experiences that foster positive relationships between all parties concerned.

We believe that interpersonal dynamics improve when physicians, nurses, and other allied health professionals, administrators, and staff learn to view each other with compassion.[8,18] This requires learning to anticipate and control the difficult interactions that come when high-powered, busy people work together. Two sorts of interventions can help here: Continuing education programs that teach about the psychology of physicians, nurses, and administrators and in-service and continuing education programs that train in the use of positive interpersonal skills.

Ideally, such educational sessions should be spaced throughout a calendar year and presented in a fashion that allows all physicians, staff, and administrators to attend. Alternatively, organizations may choose to devote a single day to intensive training. Figure 13-2 outlines a day-long curriculum that demonstrates how these topics can be addressed in a combination of joint and concurrent workshops for staff and physicians.

Keep Between-Group Dialogues Going

An often-quoted line from the movie *Godfather—Part I* sets the stage for our final recommendation: "Keep your friends close and your enemies closer."

Today's medical workplaces are complex, interpersonal systems that require ongoing diligence to recognize, prevent, or correct signs of conflict. Too often, the unhelpful "us-versus-them" mentality prevents interdisciplinary collaboration in shaping the workplace into a culture of positive interpersonal dynamics.

This problem can be prevented or corrected by regularly staging interdisciplinary problem-solving and team-building sessions. For example, some hospitals have administrators and nursing representatives from targeted hospital units meet regularly with physician representatives from the practices that serve those units. Nurses on each unit may opt to elect physicians they trust to serve as their representatives to the physicians' respective practices. This process encourages collegial repair attempts when physicians and nurses experience low-level conflict, before attitudes harden.

HOW GOOD CAN IT GET?

In earlier chapters, we listed a number of examples of how bad it can get for medical organizations when discord reins. We close with a description of the most impressive example of physician collegiality we have encountered.

We were recently invited to deliver an after-dinner address to the annual gathering of physicians and their spouses from Pinehurst Surgical Clinic, P.A., in Pinehurst, North Carolina. This is a large, multispecialty surgical group practice that has been in operation for more than 50 years. The very fact that this group would seek out a presentation on work–family balance should have cued us to the fact that it was special. But our first "this group is different" thought did not surface until the predinner social hour.

FIGURE 13-2

A Day-Long Curriculum for Shaping Positive Medical Workplace Cultures

For Staff	For Physicians
I. Controlling Yourself During Uncontrollable Times	I. Stress Management for Busy Physicians: Realistic Ways to Beat Burnout
II. How to Get Along With Physicians: What They Didn't Teach You in School	II. How to Get Along With Your Staff: What They Didn't Teach You in Medical School
III. Managing Confrontation & Conflict: When the Physician Won't Listen	III. Managing Confrontation & Conflict: If Only They'd Do What I Tell Them To Do!
IV. Joint Program for Physicians and Hospital Staff	
Beyond Conflict: How to Build Positive Relationships with Patients, Colleagues, and Loved Ones	
V. Dinner Presentation for Physicians, Administrators, and Their Significant Others	
Where Are the Heroes?	
Helping Each Other Cope at Work & Home	

The first sign that we were about to be part of a celebration of a group with remarkable levels of collegiality and collaboration was the casual comment by the group's chief financial officer that "These are great doctors and great people." Even more validating was the fact that this gentleman's wife agreed: "We moved here 5 years ago, hoping to improve our quality of life, and this has proven to be a wonderful place for my husband to complete his career. I've never seen him so happy about his work. This is a remarkable organization."

Next came unsolicited comments, like the following from several of Pinehurst Surgical's employees. A senior-level nursing supervisor said, "I've never seen or known of a group of physicians who work this well together. They have their differences, but they always work them out."

A clerical staff member commented, "One thing I respect about these doctors is that they know how to work together."

Another clerical staff member followed with, "Yes they do. Even when they disagree about something, they will keep talking about it and come to at least a temporary agreement about what to do next, and then they follow through."

Next came dinner and more casual chatting that further affirmed our impressions. We learned that the organization took seriously its commitment to maintaining high levels of teamwork and that this value was openly discussed from the outset when recruiting new physicians. We also learned that the Medical Group Management Association had recently honored Pinehurst Surgical with recognition as one of the country's leading medical organizations.

As dinner progressed, the first of what proved to be a series of brief, year-end reports by physicians who headed the group's various committees began. Scanning the agenda, we noted that the mere existence of so many committees suggested that this was a multifaceted organization with a broad base of physician leadership. In addition to the typical executive committee, Pinehurst Surgical has committees attending to information technology, hospital relations, personnel, human resources, clinical research, and many other areas. This committee structure suggested to us that, at minimum, this group tries to live up to its concise mission statement that is tactfully displayed on its letterhead:

PINEHURST SURGICAL CLINIC, P.A.
Dedicated to MEDICINE. Committed to PEOPLE.

But the best was yet to come. We noticed that, as the year-end committee presentations began, everyone seemed to actually be *listening*. Dinnertime chatter quieted. Sidebar conversations ceased. Speakers were given the courtesy of an interested audience.

Then, to a person, every one of the committee chairs was remarkably gracious and generous in specifying the contributions made by other physicians and by various staff members. Self-aggrandizement was notably absent from this group's proceedings.

As dinner ended, the group's outgoing president, Dr Malcolm Shupeck, took the podium to introduce us as the evening speakers. His comments emphasized that our presence was a small token of the gratitude Pinehurst Surgical felt for the families of each of their employees and physician partners, those same families whose support facilitated the hard and productive work of this organization.

Following our presentation, incoming group president, Clifford Long, MD, delivered the collegiality *coup de grace*. With emotion and sincerity, Dr Long responded to our notion that heroes create safe spaces for others by acknowledging the heroism of the Pinehurst Surgical organization. He spoke openly of the love that these physicians demonstrate, not only for their work and for their patients but for each other.

The privilege of this glimpse into the inner workings of this remarkable medical organization affirmed for us that, indeed, as a group, physicians are extraordinary people capable of doing most things far better than most people. Resilient medical organizations take time to build. (Pinehurst Surgical has been in existence for more than 50 years!)

But in addition to the passage of time, true collegiality and collaboration hinge on a factor that is too often omitted from our discussions in the medical marketplace, the very factor that Dr Long so eloquently addressed: Love.

Speaking of the place that love has in the corporate environment, that famous Italian "philosopher," the late Vince Lombardi, coach of the Green Bay Packers, had this to say:

"Mental toughness is humility, simplicity, spartanism, and one other—love. I don't necessarily have to like my associates, but as a man I must love them. Love is loyalty; love is teamwork; love respects the dignity of the individuals. Heart power is the strength of your corporations."[27]

CONCLUSIONS

We are not suggesting that all members of an organization must become personal friends. We are simply reminding you to honor the obvious: People are the strength of any organization. How you manage your relationships will prove to be the most powerful determiner of your resilience.

REFERENCES–CHAPTER 13

1. Goleman D. *Emotional Intelligence.* New York, NY: Bantam Books; 1995.
2. Pfifferling J-H. Managing the unmanageable: The disruptive physician. *Family Practice Management.* Nov/Dec;1997:77–92.
3. Guzzo RA, Shea GP. Group performance and intergroup relations. In: Dunnette MD, Hough LM, eds. *Handbook of Industrial and Organizational Psychology.* Palo Alto, Calif: Consulting Psychologists Press; 1992:269–313.
4. Heyworth J, Witley TW, Allison EJ, Revicki DA. Predictors of work satisfaction among SHOs during accident and emergency medicine training. *Arch Emerg Med.* 1993;10:279–288.
5. Carter AJ, West MA. Sharing the burden: Teamwork in health care settings. In: Firth-Cozens J, Payne R, eds. *Stress in Health Professionals: Psychological and Organisational Causes and Interventions.* New York, NY: John Wiley & Sons; 1999:191–202.
6. Murphy LR. Organisational interventions to reduce stress in health care professionals. In: Firth-Cozens J, Payne R, eds. *Stress in Health Professionals: Psychological and Organisational Causes and Interventions.* New York, NY: John Wiley & Sons; 1999:149–162.
7. Barnett RC, Rivers C. *She Works/He Works: How Two-Income Families are Happier, Healthier, and Better Off.* San Francisco, Calif: Harper; 1996.
8. Sotile WM, Sotile MO. Conflict management: Part 1. How to shape positive relationships in medical practices and hospitals. *The Physician Executive.* 1999;25:57–61.
9. Cooper CL, Rout U, Faragher B. Mental health, job satisfaction, and job stress among general practitioners. *BMJ.* 1989;298:366–370.
10. Lowes R. Taming the disruptive doctor. *Med Econ.* 1998;5:67–68, 73–74, 77–78, 80.
11. Right Management Consultants. *Lessons Learned from Mergers & Acquisitions: Best Practices in Workforce Integration.* Philadelphia. Pa: Right Management Consultants, Inc; 1999.
12. The Conference Board. HR challenges in mergers and acquisitions. *HR Executive Review.* 1997;5(2).
13. Sotile WM, Sotile MO. The angry physician: I. The temper-tantruming physician. *The Physician Executive.* 1996;22:30–34.
14. Sotile WM, Sotile MO. The angry physician: II. Managing yourself while managing others. *The Physician Executive.* 1996;22:39–42.

15. Harper-Neeld E. Change Awareness (workshop manual). Baton Rouge, La: Shell, Inc; 1995.
16. Ryan KD, Oestreich DK. *Driving Fear Out of the Workplace,* 2nd ed. San Francisco, Calif: Jossey-Bass; 1998.
17. Collins JC, Porras JI. *Built to Last: Successful Habits of Visionary Companies.* New York, NY: HarperCollins; 1994.
18. Sotile WM, Sotile MO. Conflict management: Part 2. How to shape positive relationships in medical practices and hospitals. *The Physician Executive.* 1999;25:51–55.
19. Wong BD. Collegiality and collaboration. Workshop presented to: American Hospital Association; 1994; New Orleans, La.
20. Baldwin PJ, Newton RW, Buckley G, Roberts MA, Dodd M. Senior house officers in medicine: Postal survey of training and work experience. *BMJ.* 1997; 314:740–743.
21. Diaz A, McMillin J. A definition and description of nurse abuse. *West J Nurs Res.* 1991;13:97–109.
22. Baron R. Countering the effects of destructive criticism: The relative efficacy of four interventions. *J Appl Psychol.* 1990;75:3.
23. Kelly R, Caplan J. How Bell Labs creates star performers. *Harvard Business Review,* July–Aug, 1993.
24. Csikszentmihalyi M. *Finding Flow.* New York, NY: Basic Books; 1997.
25. Novack DH, Suchman AL, Clark W, Epstein RM, Najberg E, Kaplan C. Calibrating the physician: Personal awareness and effective patient care. *JAMA.* 1997;278:502–509.
26. Marcus L, Dorn BC, Kritek PB, Miller VG, Wyatt JB. *Renegotiating Health Care: Resolving Conflict to Build Collaboration.* San Francisco, Calif: Jossey-Bass; 1995.
27. Peters T. *In Search of Excellence.* New York, NY: Warner, 1984.

INDEX

A

Aach, RD, 251
Abuse, medical trainees and, 255–257, 277
Accommodator management style, for conflict, 141
Accomplishment, diminished sense of, 6
Activities, categories of, 94–95
Adaptation energy, 91
Addison, RB, 280, 281
Aggression, 159
Ainsworth-Vaughn, N, 220–221
Alan, R, 167
Alcoholism, 32
Aldwin, C, 55, 57
Amik, TL, 242
Andrasik, F, 249, 265, 280, 281
Anger, 78
  controlling behavior and, 168–171
  countering physiological arousal of, 166–167
  disappointments and, 160–161
  disrupting sequences of, 165–173
  dissatisfaction and, 161
  do's and don'ts for managing, 188
  expressing, 157–159
  generators and minimizers, 170–173
  grief and, 160–161
  identifying provocations and, 166
  loss and, 160–161
  managing, 159, 167–169
  mental rehearsal for, 174
  personal effects of, 162–163
  personality scripting and, 162
  pinpointing, 160–162
  vs psychological arousal, 164–165
  recognizing three flavors of, 159
  sequence for, 156–157
  time-outs from, 173
Anxiety, 78

Arousal, emotional, 164
Aschenbrener, CA, 139
Assertiveness, communicators and, 214–215
Assessments, for stress, 32–37
Attitudes
  managing, 19–20
  removing negative, 79–80
Authority figures, conflicts with, 14, 150
Autonomy, loss of physician, 11–12
Avoidance management style, for conflict, 140
Avoidant coping, 56

B

Balance. *See* Work–life balance
Balanced life, myth of, 105–108
Baldwin, DC, 256
Barnard, S, 225
Beckman, H, 212
Being Careful coping theme, 59
Being Perfect coping theme, 58
Being Strong coping theme, 57
Benefits, withdrawal of earned, and conflict, 149
Bisexual medical trainees, 257–259
Bolden, RI, 32
Borrill, CS, 32
Brandsma, JM, 7, 54
Brittain, HM, 267
Brogan, DJ, 259
Brown, RC, 196
Brownouts, 39–40
Brunicrdi, FC, 108
Buckman, R, 216
Burke, BP, 260
Burnout, 4–6
  causes of, 6–9
  factors contributing to, 5–6
  perceived work stress and, 7–9

personality makeup and, 7
recognizing risks and symptoms of, 21–22

C

Camp, MG, 271
Career dissatisfaction, 4
Carnes, M, 131
Carter, AJ, 32, 294
Carter, JD, 40–42
Carter, JM, 40–42
Carver, C, 82
Casale, H, 191–192
Chambre, KM, 258
Change. *See also* Coping; Pattern disruption
    accepting, 77, 234–235
    being realistic about stress of, 231–232
    helping others to cope with, 241–244
    maintaining control and, 233–234
    operationalizing worries about, 238–239
    as opportunity, 239
    types of, 235–238
    understanding processes of, 240–241
Choices, making self-protective, 20
Clair, DK, 267
Classen, DC, 280
Codes of conduct, 198–199
Cognitive reframing strategies, for painful emotions, 80
Collaboration
    management style, for conflict, 141
    in mature medical organizations, 311–312
Collegiality
    lack of, and physicians, 17
    in mature medical organizations, 311–312
Collins, JC, 307
Communication
    with colleagues, 212
    with loved ones, 212–213
    with patients, 211–212
    poor, and conflict, 149–150

Communicators
    assertiveness and, 214–215
    being specific and, 223–224
    characteristics of good, 213–214
    conveying warmth and, 215–216
    discretion and, 224
    empathy and, 216–219
    humor and, 225
    listening and, 219–223
    speaking pace of, 225–226
    use of positive words by, 225
Compromiser management style, for conflict, 140–141
Compulsive working, and work addiction, 40–43
Conflict. *See also* Negotiation
    accommodator management style, 141
    avoider management style, 140
    collaborator management style, 141
    compromiser management style, 140–141
    criticism as source of, 147–148
    definition of, 177–178
    dominator management style, 139
    feedback for correcting, 151–152
    guidelines for negotiating, 182–187
    lack of teamwork and, 148–149
    lack of training, and, 148
    lack of trust and, 149
    in medical workplaces, 146–150
    preventing, 150
    as problem *vs* opportunity, 178
    resolving, 135–136
    scale for stages of, 144–146
    superiors and, 14, 150
Conflict Scale, Stages of, 144–146
Confrontations, guidelines for, 202–206
Continuous change, 237
Contracts, psychological, 10
Control, loss of, and coping, 233
Coombs, RH, 249, 257
Cooney, TG, 251
Cooper, CI, 31
Cooper, RK, 92
Coping. *See also* Change
    control and, 233–234
    emotion-focused, 56